Hair Rules!

Hair Rules!

The Ultimate Hair-Care Guide for Women
with Kinky, Curly, or Wavy Hair

A. Dickey

Foreword by Tomiko Fraser

Introduction by Louis Licari

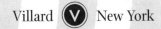
Villard Ⓥ New York

LIBRARY OF CONGRESS CATALOGING-IN-PUBLICATION DATA
Dickey, A.
   Hair rules! : the ultimate hair-care guide for women with kinky, curly, or wavy hair / A. Dickey; foreword by Tomiko Fraser; introduction by Louis Licari.
      p.   cm.
   ISBN 0-375-76130-6 (pbk.)
      1. Hair—Care and hygiene.   I. Title.

RL91 .D535 2003
646.7'24—dc21   2002191067

Villard Books website address: www.villard.com
Printed in the United States of America
9 8 7 6 5 4 3 2

First Edition

BOOK DESIGN BY MERCEDES EVERETT

This book is dedicated to my grandparents

Mac and Daisy Dickey

Foreword

Tomiko Fraser

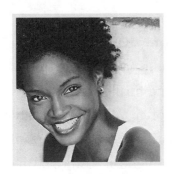

My hair. My hair has been a topic of conversation for as long as I can remember. It started with my entry into this world and the inevitable question on all black folks' minds when a black girl is born: "Does she have *good* hair?" Sitting in front of my mother's stove as a young girl while she straightened my hair (and I'd better not move or else I'd get the burn of my life). Going on long bus trips as a teenager to a faraway beauty salon—I still don't know why we had to travel so far—to have my hair relaxed. I would leave the salon smelling of hair products and feeling the breeze finally reach my freshly relaxed scalp. (Don't act like you don't know what I'm talking about.) My hair has always been, first and foremost, an undertaking.

Fast-forward to my new career as a model. I had arrived! I just knew that I would be in good hands because the people whom I worked with were professionals. Right? I quickly learned that just because someone had a portfolio full of famous women whose hair they'd got their hands on didn't mean that all was safe and sound. If I began to tell you all of the horror stories about how my hair was fried, twisted, pulled, colored, weaved, wigged, and so on, your head would spin. Needless to say, it wasn't always cute. I longed for the day when I could look in the mirror and be happy with what had been done to my poor little head. I even got to the point where I would bring all my own tools to ensure a satisfactory job. I carried wigs, hairpieces, products, combs, brushes, curling irons, straightening combs . . . the list goes on. I have made many a hairstylist green with envy because of my collection of materials. (They didn't understand that a girl's gotta do what a girl's gotta do.)

So, it should come as no surprise to you that my hair was a constant source of stress for me. I just didn't believe that the so-called professionals or I would ever get it right. That constant worrying finally led to what is affectionately called a "stress spot" on the top of my head. (Basically, ladies, I had a bald spot.) I attribute it to a combination of worry and plain old wear and tear. My poor little head had had enough. It wasn't playing by my rules anymore. It had developed a mind of its own. There was nothing I could do. I tried letting my natural hair grow in, only to have it break off again once I relaxed it. I wore a weave for a few years, hoping that the hair would regrow, to no avail. I even sported an old man's comb-over for a short period of time. It was sad. Really sad. (It's okay to laugh because I sure do. *Now.*)

Enter Mr. Dickey. Dickey was, throughout all my hair drama, the sole voice of reason. "Girl, you know you need to wear your hair natural" was his mantra. He'd been a world-renowned hairstylist for many years, so I guess he felt like he knew something. But he was dealing with *my* hair. I knew what worked for me. Right? How was he going to tell someone in my position, with my level of visibility, to wear a natural? Didn't he know that I had worked long and hard to establish my look? When clients asked for Tomiko, they knew they were getting "the black girl next door." I couldn't jeopardize that with a big ole 'fro! What was he thinking? The nerve!

So, he did as I asked and relaxed, straightened, or weaved my hair. Well, wouldn't you know it? My stress spot grew even larger. And this time with a vengeance! I remember sitting on the bathroom floor of a bed-and-breakfast, where I was spending the weekend a few years ago, with my hair *coming out in my hands!!* That's it! Time out! This had gotten ridiculous!

Guess where I was that Monday morning? In Dickey's chair getting all of my relaxed hair cut off. "*Off,*" I said. I cried like a baby. And he wasn't all gentle and sweet. He cut my hair off like it had just slapped him in the face. He was finally getting his way. I couldn't bear to look in the mirror. Who was this person? And why was she bald-headed? I didn't want to look at her anymore. So, I quickly left the salon with my head hanging low.

The story doesn't end there, folks. For the record, I am the zodiac sign that is often accused of being quite stubborn. So, as soon as my hair grew back, I found a different hairstylist to relax it for me. Dickey would not be right if I had my way. Let's just jump ahead here—BALD-HEADED MODEL SEEN RUNNING AND SCREAMING DOWN FIFTH AVENUE WITH HANDS FULL OF HER OWN HAIR! Done. Over. The fat lady had sung. I knew what I needed to do.

After much consulting with friends, family, agents, passersby on the street, etc., I decided it was time to let my hair do what it wanted to do: live in its natural state. (Isn't that all we really want anyway?) The final test came when my agents had to contact the execs at Maybelline (with whom I had a cosmetics campaign—the first African-American woman to do so with the cosmetics giant, I might add). I had appeased them for several years with various numbers of weaves. They wanted long, cascading curls, they got it. They wanted bone-straight, Asian-looking hair, they got it. Hell, if they wanted me to sport a blond wig while dancing the hokey-pokey, I would have given them that, too. But, surprisingly, they were cool with my decision to wear my hair natural. They wanted me to be happy. A happy model sells lots and lots of makeup.

So here I am today, two years later, with a headful of healthy, happy, natural hair. I am thrilled! Not only am I happy, but my clients, friends, family, agents, and, most important, Dickey are happy. It seems that not only was the world ready for (gasp!) a black model with natural hair, but I was ready for them.

Dickey is offering a much-needed reminder with *Hair Rules!* Work with what you have—it's fabulous! I am so pleased that I finally listened to him and did what needed to be done years ago. Any woman with "nonconventional" (or the less politically correct terms such as nappy, kinky, coarse, etc.) hair can relate to my story. Yes, the facts may not be identical, but the drama is all the same. Dickey has answers. He doesn't just tell you what you want to hear, he gives it to you straight. No chaser. Just beautiful results. Listen to him, ladies. He knows of what he speaks.

Thank you, Dickey. For always being in my hair corner. Keep doing your thing. You are a blessing to all of the nappy-haired girls of the world. I love you.

Contents

Introduction

Louis Licari

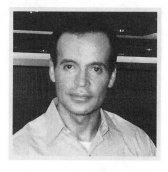

When Dickey asked me to write the introduction to *Hair Rules!* I realized how much need there was for this book. Kinky and curly hair are different from straight hair. They are often drier, and they require different styling techniques and styling products, and a gentler hand when you are coloring them. They also require more expertise than straight hair does to care for and style. Nonstraight hair often needs multiple chemical services: It is not unusual for a woman with this type of hair to relax her hair and then want to try hair color. This requires the know-how of when and how these different services should be done.

There seems to be a general lack of information about kinky and curly hair. Women of color and all other women with nonstraight hair have been left out of the loop when it comes to obtaining great-looking hair. Industry insiders often shy away from nonstraight hair because of their own ignorance. They seem to regard kinky and curly hair as being too complicated for the nonprofessional. And yet, these types of hair are beautiful and actually easy to care for.

Dickey's book addresses these issues head-on. (Please forgive my pun.) It's time for you to learn all of his expert tips, gleaned from years of experience styling the hair of the world's most famous and beautiful women. This is Dickey's insider's guide to great-looking hair with little effort. He tells all the dos and don'ts for maintaining healthy hair. He explains hairstyling trends, weaves, and relaxing techniques, and shares his considerable experience on how to do all these procedures safely without bias against any one look.

It is time to be proud of and love your nonstraight hair. Your years of frustration and hate are over. All your hair's secrets and mysteries are exposed. *Hair Rules!* has arrived.

Hair Rules!

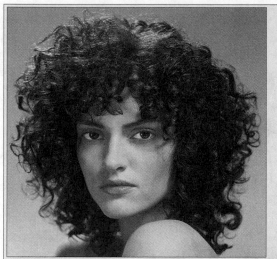
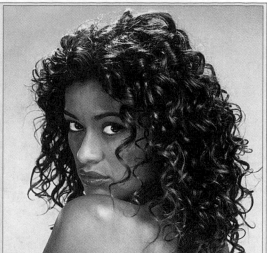
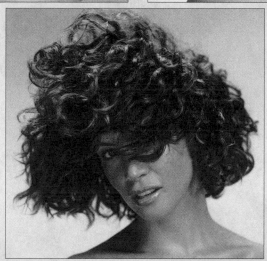
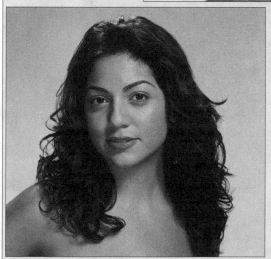
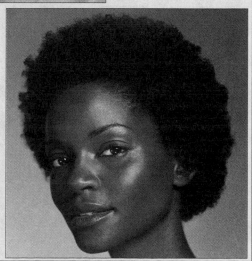

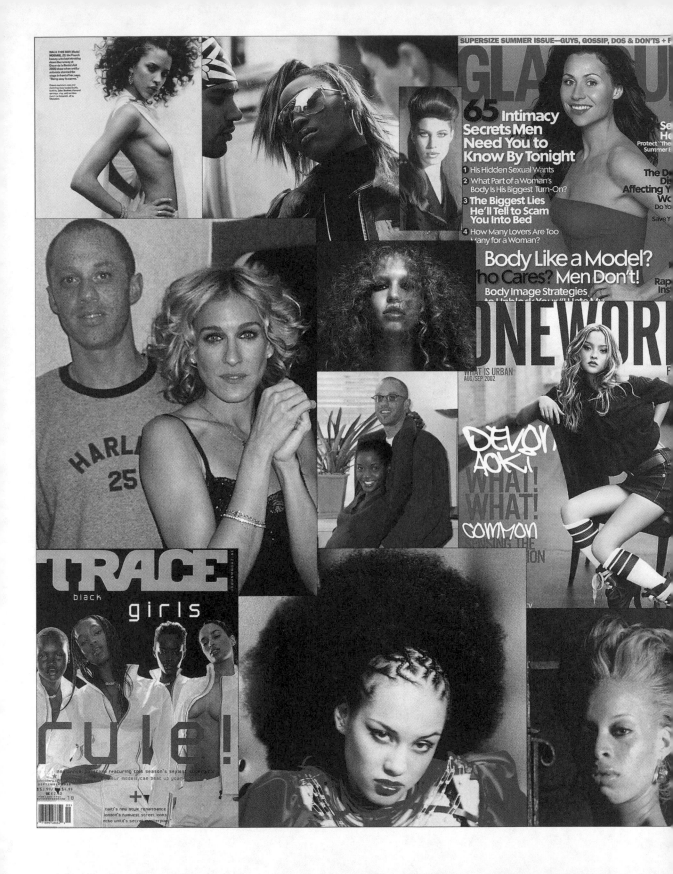

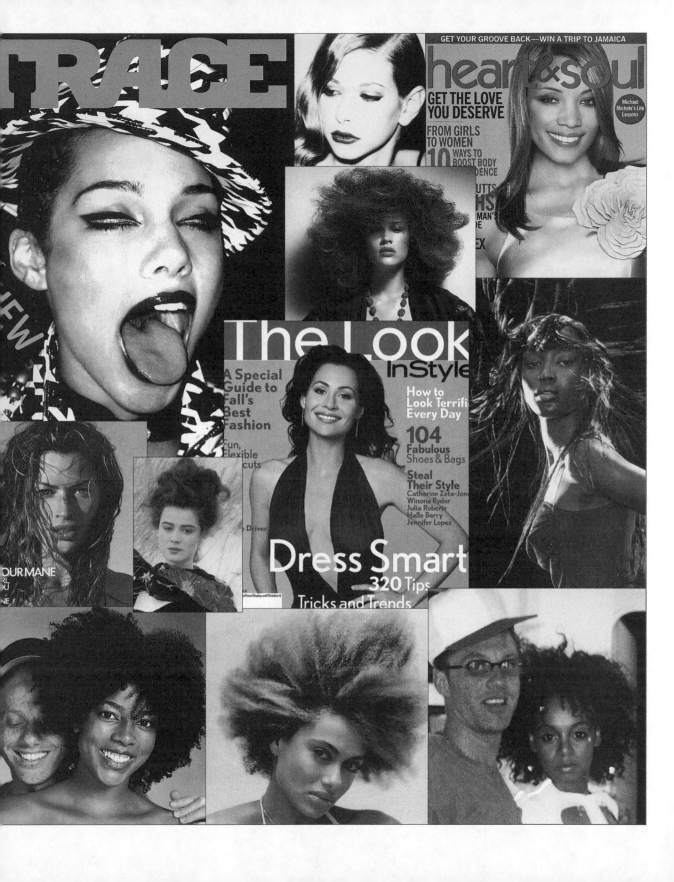

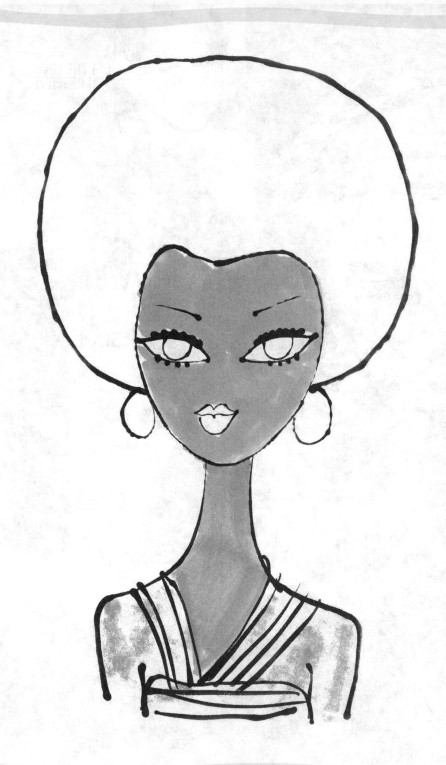

Chapter 1

Hairitage

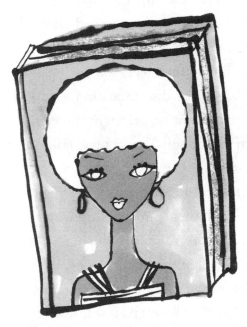

Your "Hairitage," or a Little History of Nonstraight Hair

It is only in the past thirty years that hair that is other than straight has been admired by America's mainstream culture. Even so, women with nonstraight hair, i.e., women of color, Jewish women, and women of mixed ancestry, still retain negative beliefs about their hair. Among the most prevalent of these beliefs is one that says straight hair is inherently better than kinky, curly, or wavy hair. In other words, straight hair is "good" and other textures are "bad." We continue to think of silky, straight hair as easy to comb, volumeless, and requiring little or no maintenance. (The grass is always greener . . .) Just in case you fast-forwarded past the Introduction, I'll repeat myself here: There is really no such thing as good hair or bad hair. It doesn't matter what kind of hair you have. If I were to make any distinction, after years as a professional stylist, it would be between a healthy head of hair and an unhealthy head of hair. In my practice, that is what really determines good or bad hair. And healthy hair trumps all textures and types!

In the early 1970s, women of all races gloried in their natural hair texture. Self-pride flourished during that liberating, self-expressive time. By the late 1970s, however, the hair and cosmetic companies, having lost money, began an assault on the psyches of women and embarked on extensive advertising campaigns lionizing conservative, straight-haired styles. Their success, a return to the primacy of straightened hair, was accompanied by an even more disturbing trend: workplace discrimination against women of color who wore naturals or braids. Not surprisingly, the right to wear one's clean, coiffed hair in an attractive, non-Eurocentric fashion had to be fought for all the way to the Supreme Court.

In any battle there are casualties, as there were for the victors of hairstyle choice. Many ambitious professional women remained convinced that their career mobility would be eclipsed if they didn't conform to European standards of hair beauty. To this day, when women in high-profile positions go into a meeting with straight, styled hair, it may be because they feel more put together and secure that they'll be taken seriously by their male counterparts. I'll be the first to admit that there is truth to that: Straight hair can convey a stern, no-nonsense, dare I say "I-can-be-a-bitch-if-I-have-to" look. The same reservations about career mobility hold true for black women and braids in the workplace. It has only been since the 1990s that professional women of color have sported braids.

With this second wave of liberation, I thought it was high time for *Hair Rules!* My mission is simple: to advise and encourage *all* women with nonstraight hair to strive to attain their beauty, whatever their ethnicity, and whatever their tastes.

With the tide turning toward more inclusiveness and variety, the beauty and cosmetics industry has done an about-face and developed some highly innovative, chemically altering products that are much safer and less damaging than ever before. Despite these advances, for those of you who are victims of hair hatred, there's no telling what you'll do if it were left up to you! One of the most important things you *can* do is to recognize why it is you want to change your hair. Once you've deduced that, and it's on a positive tip—"I want a more professional look," or "I've changed," or "I know I'll look better with longer hair"—then the sky's the limit.

Knowing your own hair texture and the current state of your hair is the next step in realizing what styling options you have. The texture and condition of your hair should determine the boundaries of what you can do. Before your shoulders slump, hang on! The boundaries are wider and far more exciting than you would imagine. For now, put away the fashion and hair magazines. Get honest with yourself and the hair that's on your head. All of our society's misconceptions and the media's mixed-message images (not to mention those of self-interested stylists) that trickle down to you will only frustrate and confuse you. It's time you knew your true "hairitage."

Your Texture, Your Type

Okay, I've stopped preaching (for now)! Let's get down to business. Nonstraight hair ranges from kinky, the curliest, to wavy, which is slightly less curly, and everything in between. For humans as a species, there are few actual differences among people. Hair is one of them. Most people who populate the Earth have the kinds of kinky, curly, or wavy hair I'm writing about. So, you're part of a big club.

All hair, whether straight, wavy, curly, or kinky, is comprised of two essential parts: the root, which is the structure beneath the skin surface, and the hair shaft (or stem), which extends above the skin surface. The hair shaft itself is made of three parts—the *medulla,* the *cortex,* and the *cuticle.* If you cut one of your own hairs and placed it under a microscope, its cross-section would reveal distinctive cellular "sleeves" that make up your hair. The innermost core of the shaft, the medulla, contains melanin granules, which determine our God-given hair color. The next "sleeve" is the cortex, which is actually the thickest part of the shaft. It is the cortex that determines hair's strength, resilience, and moisture content.

The cuticle is what we see and think of as our hair. It is made up of overlapping keratin (protein) cells that lie closely on the shaft like fish scales. Cuticles have between seven to ten layers. (The number of layers determines the diameter of an individual hair.) Healthy hair is defined by a person's having an intact cuticle. On the other hand, damaged hair, whether the damage comes from heat, brushing, or chemical processing, is defined as hair having a cuticle whose "scales" have lifted, separated, or broken away from the shaft. Once a hair's cortex and medulla are exposed, the hair is susceptible to breakage.

While it is the hair shaft that most of us are concerned about (and are willing to spend big bucks on), the fact is that it is the humble, invisible root that is connected to a blood supply and oil glands. (This is my way of telling you that your health directly affects your hair.) The truth is that, while I don't want to bore you with the anatomy of hair, I do want you to remember that though the hair shaft doesn't have nerve endings (which is why getting a haircut isn't classified as major surgery, no matter what you think), it is attached to the root. What happens to your roots (connected as they are to blood vessels and oil glands) has much to do with the condition of each and every hair shaft.

When we use terms like straight, wavy, curly, and kinky, we are talking about the configuration, or shape, of each hair. Let's call that shape hair *type.* Hair type is determined by the *follicle,* the scalp indentation that houses the root. Thanks to genetics, follicles vary in size, shape, and thickness. Whatever size, shape, and thickness your follicles are determine your hair shape and, hence, type. All hair types come in three major *textures*— coarse, medium, and fine. (Incidentally, you can have a combination of all three on different parts of your head. Hair grows at a rate of approximately a quarter to a half inch per month, and this new growth can arrive in any texture.) In addition to texture, we tend to classify hair's volume using terms like thick and thin, or *fine.* It can be somewhat confusing because it's not the individual diameter of each hair that determines whether you have thick or fine hair, it's the number of shafts per square inch. So, you may very well have coarse hair, but not a lot of it, and be classified as having fine hair—just as you can have fine hair and tons of it, yet be classified as having thick hair. See how easily one can get mixed up?

As you can see, hair itself is complex and amazing. Whole chapters could be written on the various classifications. For you, though, it's your type and texture that determine your styling options, and how you can best care for your hair. Let me explain the major types of hair:

- Coiled-kinky hair, which most of you know as kinky hair, is related to curly hair in that it is very tightly coiled and curled together. (Despite the way many of you mistreat your kinky hair, this stuff is extremely fragile! Remember, the more coiled the hair shaft, the more fragile the hair.) Contrary to the popular belief that all kinky hair is coarse, it, too, can be fine- or medium-textured. Regardless of texture, kinky hair has lots and lots of densely packed thin strands. Kinky hair is distinguished by its lack of shine, but it is capable of having a beautiful luster and sheen if it's healthy.

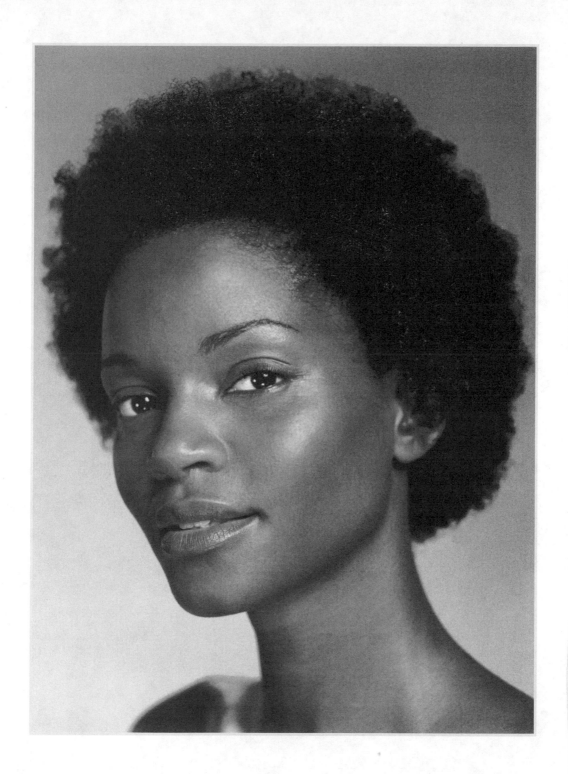

*There is really no such thing as
good hair or bad hair. Healthy hair
trumps all textures and types.*

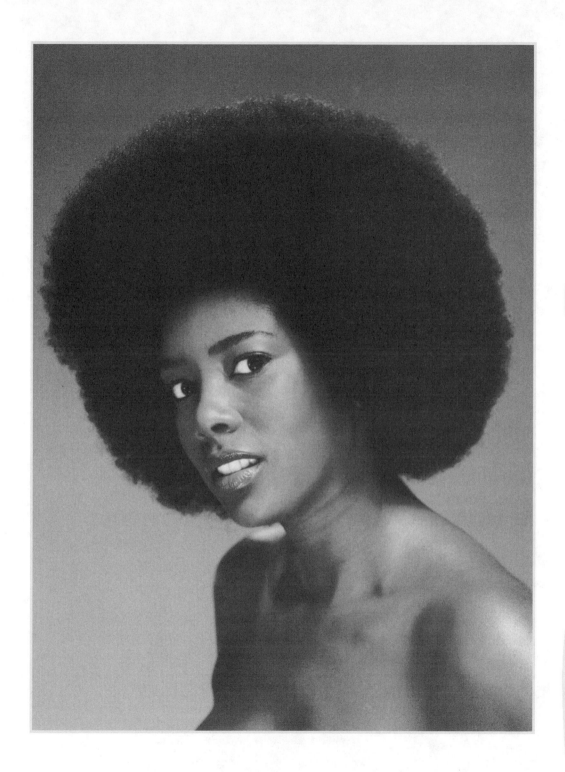

- Curly hair has a looped S-pattern, a coil, because the cuticle layers don't lie down as flat as those of wavy hair. Curly hair, too, can be fine, medium, or coarse textured. It has less shine than wavy hair does, and a considerable amount of luster. The curlier your natural hair is, the less the cuticles lie down. In order to straighten curly hair, you have to smooth down and flatten the cuticle with heat. The smoother the surface, the shinier the surface.

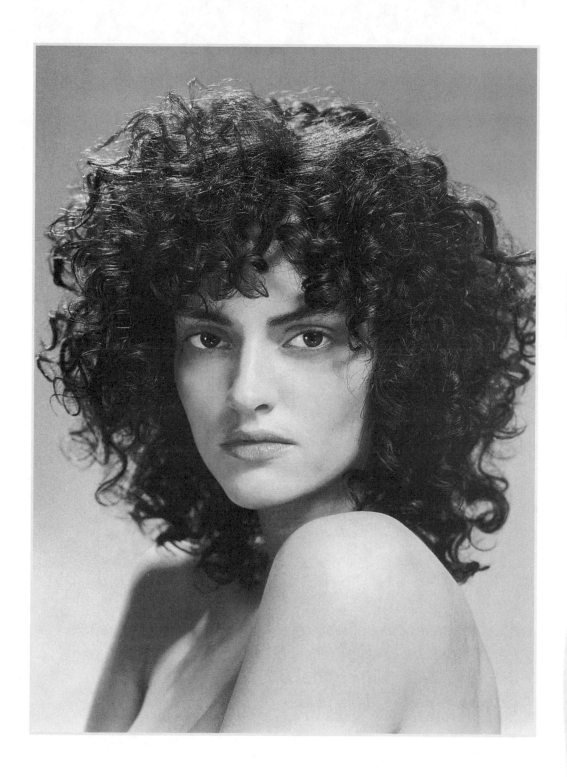

*Most people who populate the
Earth have the kinds of kinky, curly,
or wavy hair I'm writing about.
So, you're part of a big club.*

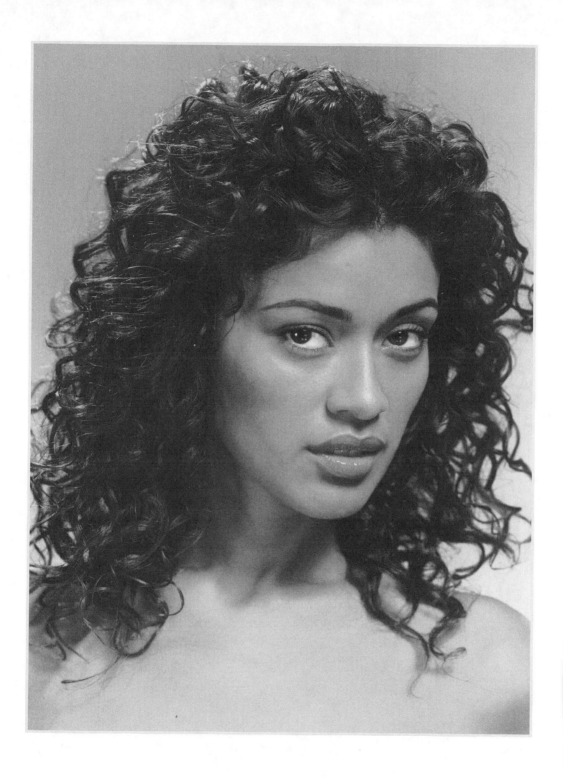

- Wavy hair has a definite S-pattern to it. Its cuticle lies almost flat, giving the hair some shine. Wavy hair can be fine, medium, or coarse textured.

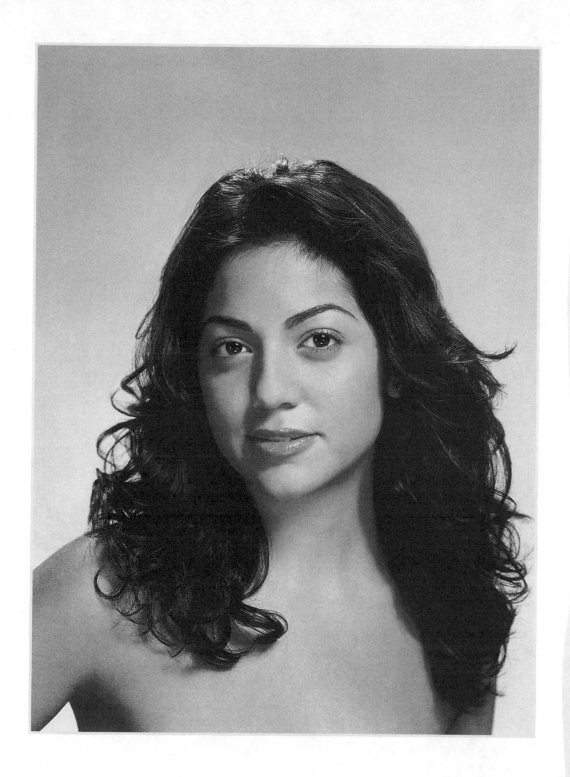

Nonstraight hair ranges from kinky, the curliest, to wavy, which is slightly less curly, and everything in between.

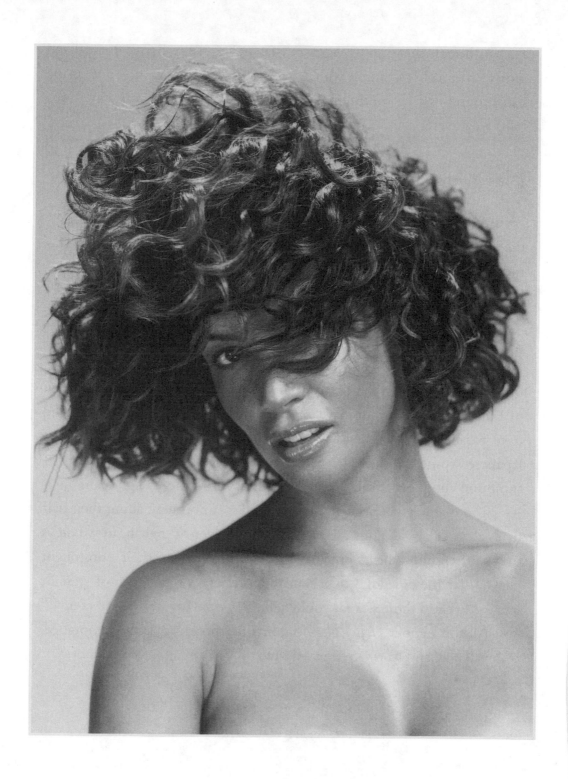

Although there isn't a hard-and-fast relationship between type and glossiness, a rule of thumb would be that straight hair shines, and as the hair progresses on a continuum through wavy all the way to kinky it obtains a characteristic we call luster.

Hair Myths

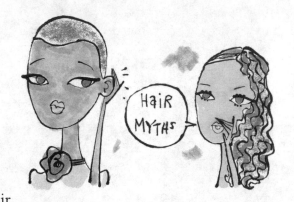

Living in a nation that has the northern European model as its standard of hair beauty, many African-American women have legitimate issues about their hair. Yet, they are not alone, which is why this book was written for *all* women with nonstraight hair. Many women of European ancestry also have extremely wavy, curly, or kinky hair, and have parallel issues about theirs. It's a big and complex world: I've met Japanese women with kinky hair. Meeting them shattered my own assumption about genetically "pure" Asians having bone-straight hair.

Too many women are walking around so ambivalent about their hair that they neglect it. They are cheating themselves of their beauty. Bad as that is, there are other women who out-and-out hate their nonstraight hair. What they've done to it (and themselves) for the sake of straight hair . . . well, if those strands could talk, they'd be crying, "Have mercy!"

All throughout *Hair Rules!* I will refute those myths that ignorance, ambivalence, and hair hatred have spawned.

•　　　•　　　•

Choosing a Good Stylist

A woman can pick a good stylist anywhere if she has sufficient knowledge about her own hair. This is important for today's woman, who has as much going on as any man, yet must still be concerned about her appearance. My advice and suggestions make it possible for a busy, multitasking person such as yourself to feel confident choosing a good stylist at home and away. In today's fast-paced world, the maintenance required to look your best is quite a commitment. Finding a stylist to help maintain your hair is an important first step. Convenience; a nice, clean atmosphere; and someone who is as concerned about your hair as you are and respects your time are some of the things you should look for when choosing a hairstylist.

Consider the way you think about eating out. If you are a good cook, when you eat out you want a place that serves the food you love, prepared by a chef who is as good a cook as you are, if not better. Not only that, if you have told your waiter that you don't eat shellfish, why would you pay good money when he brings you a plate of unwashed, undercooked mussels drowned in reconstituted lemon juice? It's really not much different when choosing a hairstylist. This is someone in whom you should feel absolute confidence that she or he can do things for and to your hair that are as good as or better than you can do yourself. Now that you are armed with knowledge about hair anatomy, type, and texture, does it make any sense to set aside time in your schedule for someone who can't "take your order" based on your preferences, tastes, and educated knowledge about your hair, as well as your lifestyle and age?

Your instincts are going to direct you to someone whose work you've seen and liked. Providing she or he is available, the next thing you need to find out is whether or not the stylist really listens to what you're asking for. That, of course, doesn't mean what you want is what you'll get, given your hair's condition, its texture, your lifestyle and age, but a good stylist will try to accommodate your wishes while he or she uses her professional expertise to maximize your looks. Please be honest with yourself before you walk into that salon and get some hairstylist to believe all your drama! You might walk out looking like Ms. Whodunit!

Any good stylist will tell you word-of-mouth is the best form of advertising. If you find yourself complimenting someone's cut or style, then, by all means, ask for the source. Once you've identified a particular stylist, call and find out if an appointment is necessary for an initial consultation. Even if an appointment isn't necessary, don't settle for a phone conversation. No reputable stylist will consult over the phone about a head of hair he or she can't see! There's usually no charge for a consultation, but keep your questions to a minimum. Time is money, and courtesy dictates that you not take more than ten or fifteen minutes of the stylist's time.

If you live in or near a large city, another excellent way of finding a stylist is by browsing through beauty and fashion magazines. (Remember, I said put them away, not throw them away!) A lot of the magazines have credits that list hairstylists who work both for the magazine and in a nearby salon.

Questions to ask the stylist? Depending on the general condition of your hair, you should expect to receive honest answers about your current or desired hairstyle. Questions that are important to ask are: What type of products do you use and what type of services do you provide? What are your hours? Do you work on all types and textures? How long have you been a hairstylist? In other words, ask about everything except the stylist's fees. For most stylists, that matter is best discussed with the salon's receptionist. Hairstylists are artists; the commerce is handled by a salon's front-desk staff.

Reform and Rehabilitation (R&R)

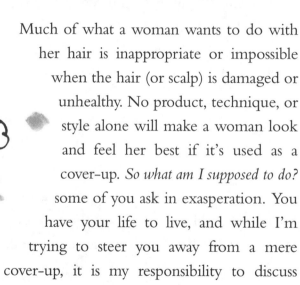

Much of what a woman wants to do with her hair is inappropriate or impossible when the hair (or scalp) is damaged or unhealthy. No product, technique, or style alone will make a woman look and feel her best if it's used as a cover-up. *So what am I supposed to do?* some of you ask in exasperation. You have your life to live, and while I'm trying to steer you away from a mere cover-up, it is my responsibility to discuss what your options are as your hair goes through a convalescence. Of course you're going to need some expert help.

If you find that your hair is in need of R&R (just as some of you suspected all along), I recommend that in addition to reading this chapter, you might also read Chapter 8, "The Doctor Can See You Now." It is full of pertinent information about what to do (and not do) when your hair and scalp have been damaged. There's a very good chance that your hair didn't get to its damaged state without some help, and it won't be restored without some help. It may be time for you to learn how to choose a competent stylist.

For you, the most important work is to restore your hair to its original beauty before you dive wholeheartedly into the world of permanently altering your texture and/or color, which *Hair Rules!* explores in later chapters. It's not that those things won't be available to you, it's just that (and again, your having healthy hair is my number-one priority) without hair that can withstand the stresses of man-made beautification, none of the products, services, or techniques I'll be discussing will enhance your beauty in lasting ways. And that's what we want, don't we? So, take heart, and read on!

It would be unethical for me to suggest a detailed regimen of R&R in this book. After all, I haven't seen you. But don't ever think of yourself as a hopeless case. Whenever your hair has reached a 911 state of emergency, the best and wisest course of action is to stop whatever treatments or styling options you've been habitually using and make an appointment with a dermatologist for a consultation.

When you're thinking of seeking professional help, be prepared to accurately and honestly discuss the state of your hair. You should be able to explain the details of your cleaning, conditioning, and styling routines, and even some details about your lifestyle. (I'm sure you know that age, diet, environment, and hair-care products and treatments all have an effect on your hair. That's why it's important that you freely share this information.) The dermatologist may ask:

— What shampoos and conditioners do you use?
— What styling products and appliances do you use?

— Have you ever colored or do you color your hair?

— Have you ever permed or do you perm your hair?

— How often do you shampoo?

— How often do you condition your hair?

— Have you worn or do you wear hair additions?

— How often do you have your hair cut or trimmed?

— Have there been any important life changes that have caused you positive or negative stress, such as pregnancy, a new marriage, a divorce, job changes, deaths, or any other major event?

It might be a good idea to take a moment to jot down the answers to these questions. Often, we don't give any thought to what's going on in our life until we force ourselves to recall it. Now, I'm not saying that the kind of care and treatment you might need can be easily determined by asking yourself a few questions in the privacy of your home. But I do know that considering these questions puts you in a frame of mind to speak knowledgeably with a dermatologist when you do have your initial meeting.

The dermatologist may test your hair and scalp and recommend a course of treatment, or may refer you to a stylist or a trichologist, an experienced hairdresser who specializes in working on abnormal hair and scalp conditions.

Much of the advice and guidance from the previous section, "Choosing a Good Stylist," applies when you begin the process of repairing damage done to your hair and scalp. Not only can skilled professionals work with you to "recover" your hair, they can suggest a number of appropriate options while your hair and scalp are undergoing rehabilitation so that you can maintain an attractive appearance that complements your lifestyle. For those of you who need R&R, it's important to get a couple of recommendations from people who have been clients of a particular stylist or trichologist. After all, this is someone with whom you'll be working intimately, and he or she will become part nurse, part therapist, and part magician.

If it's been determined that emotional stress is a significant factor in your hair's condition, seek counseling or get some exercise on a regular basis. (See Dr. Downie's remarks in Chapter 8 about the role stress plays in treatment outcomes.) Incorporating exercise or therapeutic counseling into one's life may become as important as medications toward restoring your hair and scalp to optimal health. One of the reasons a reputable hair professional won't treat a hair condition indefinitely is that if underlying causes are not addressed, no amount of treatment with oral medications or topical ointments is going to make a noticeable and lasting change.

When damage to your hair or scalp is the result of chemicals or heat, you should be prepared for a long partnership with your hair professional. With cooperative diligence and patience, the detrimental effects to your hair and scalp can be lessened, and sometimes reversed.

Let me say up front that it takes no small courage to face up to hair damage. I think this is particularly true when you realize that you are responsible for what has happened to your hair. But what about all of you who were doing the right thing and your hair's still in trouble? You never did your own perming, pressing, or coloring, you say. You were religious about your Saturday-morning appointment at Salon Fab-U-Lous, and have had the same hairdresser for years, you say. Unfortunately, some of the nicest, sweetest folks in the business can be incompetent or lazy. There are hairdressers who haven't kept up with the latest science in hair care. When that happens, neither you nor your hair is getting the benefit of better, safer products. Don't make me say it—but I will: There are hairdressers who just don't have any respect for nonstraight hair. (I see this all the time.)

Whatever the case may be, I have one piece of advice: *Run, don't walk* away from that person. Don't let loyalty, habit, trendiness, convenience, or nice-girls-don't-complain syndrome keep you in that chair until you are completely bald! And if you think I'm playing, call a cosmetic surgeon's office and find out just how much a hair transplant costs. 'Nuff said!

Questions & Answers

Q: Is there some type of chart that tells me what to do with my exact hair type? I'm Jewish, with curly hair that's basically all one length. How long can I go with my face shape, which is oval?

A: Determining one's *exact* hair type doesn't necessarily lead you to make better styling choices. You probably already know your type—very curly with the potential to frizz. Even if you typed your hair as thick, medium, or fine, the bottom line is that as long as you're not drying it out by too-frequent shampooing, and as long as you're using a liberal amount of conditioner each time you wash your hair, then you'll be doing right by your type.

As far as your hairstyle, I'm going to assume you wear your

hair one length because it helps to keep it from getting big. In other words, your particular cut helps to weigh down your hair. With that in mind, I'd say that layers might not be a bad idea as long as they're below the chin in front, and along the bottom only. You just want to add some movement.

Q: My hair is kinky and dry and has no shine to it. I like my cut, but my hair's so coarse. What can I do?

A: Try this simple preshampoo treatment: apply castor oil, shea butter, or olive oil to your hair, then sit under a hood dryer for ten to fifteen minutes. Afterward, shampoo out the treatment, followed by a reconditioning (using your regular conditioner). Last, apply a light essential oil like jojoba or almond oil. The point is that your hair needs as much oil and moisture as it can possibly get. Because of the nature of kinky hair, it takes a conscious effort on your part to get oil all the way to your ends. This treatment just helps it along. I guarantee you, not only will your hair feel and look beautiful, but frankly, you'll smell good enough to eat!

Q: I love my stylist and what he does for my hair, but he's never on time for me, and I get so pissed. Should I say something to him?

A: How late is he, really? Suppose you've been waiting for a half hour or less. Let's say you see your physician for your annual physical and then you decide that you have specific issues to discuss; your stylist's previous client may have occupied him in much the same way. Or, it may be that another client was a half hour late. In either instance, the courtesy your stylist extended to them would undoubtedly be extended to you. So, be gracious and thankful that when it's your turn, he's willing to spend an hour with you once you do get to see him. Add it up. An hour and a half for the sake of beauty is not too much to ask!

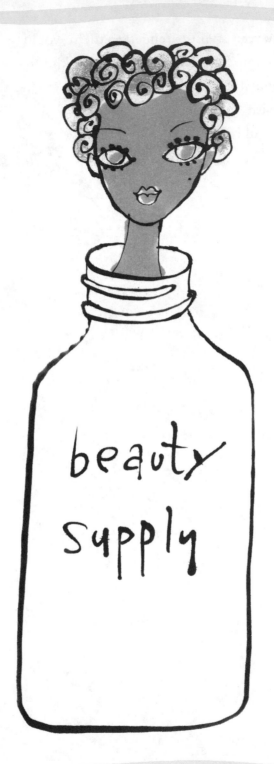

Chapter 2

Beauty Supply

So Many Products, So Little Time . . .

As I mentioned in Chapter 1, one error that even a smart and informed multitasking woman can make is to use the wrong products on her hair. With so many products on the market, it's confusing for anyone trying to decide what to purchase. How could any sensible woman not be baffled by the cornucopia of choices now available, thanks to some savvy marketing on the part of the major cosmetic companies? With all that coming at you, how can you make appropriate choices? Understanding your hair type and not pushing it beyond its limits is the critical first step. In no time, it will become easy for you to select the products that will make your hair look its best.

Despite the fact that you've known your head of hair for years, many of you still aren't certain which shampoos, conditioners, and treatments work best for your kind of hair. In this chapter of *Hair Rules!* I want to introduce you to the various products that work best with nonstraight hair. We will focus on the basics: what to use to wash and condition your hair, and using man-made and natural products for optimal maintenance and styling. First, let me ask you a question before we turn on the water. . . .

Are You a Product Junkie?

Well, are you? Do you practically have an orgasm when you enter the hair aisle of your favorite drugstore, or are you the one who can never walk by any beauty-supply store without going in and coming out with a little somethin'-somethin' in a colorful tube or jar? A product junkie can never seem to find the magical combination of products that will make her hair look like that of (insert your favorite celebrity here), even though she spends her time endlessly searching for it, especially if it claims to be a combination curl-enhancing defrizzer with a straightening balm that contains plenty of flattening serum while cleaning and conditioning. There's no such thing, you say? And yet, if I offered you a 6.5-ounce tube with those very buzzwords on it for a mere $24.99, I bet you'd thank me!

Such is the concern, even desperation, that some of you might have for your hair, that you'll try almost anything based on a promise and an alluring photo. How many times have you seen a model on TV or on a box and been seduced into purchasing and using an inappropriate product for your hair? (I can just see that bottle with the fine print ". . . for blondes only" pushed to the back of your medicine chest.) I bet you didn't know that the model you so admire spent hours being styled by a professional. I promise you that the stylist didn't use the product being advertised, since she has her own personal stash of tried-and-true products. To add insult to injury, every hair on that model's head is being attended to with each click of the camera. Is it any wonder the results differ? So, there you have it. You've been had!

The big cosmetic companies are getting hip to the spending power of minority women. (It's been said that minority women—that means many of you—account for 60 percent of hair-care sales.) In the pursuit of minority dollars the big companies are not only integrating their product sections in some stores, but—peace, be still—where the products are separate, the ethnic product section is increasing in size. The large companies are formulating products as fast as they can for this lucrative market that you've made. They just have to know what's hot!

In the last several years beauty-supply stores, too, have become more savvy and consumer-friendly. Beauty-supply owners, like the cosmetic companies, have finally awakened to the power of consumer spending. In the past, these stores used to be a big secret, a haven for pros only. Now store owners know that smart women demand to achieve the same looks for less by doing it themselves, or owning, for instance, the same flat iron as their hairdresser. (I look forward to the day that I'm shopping at my favorite beauty-supply store and run into one of my clients!) While the large companies and the supply stores have responded to your demands, offering more choice and better, more convenient products, sometimes you can leave a store with more product than you need. Often it's because you're buying the brand name, and not the product that works best for your hair type.

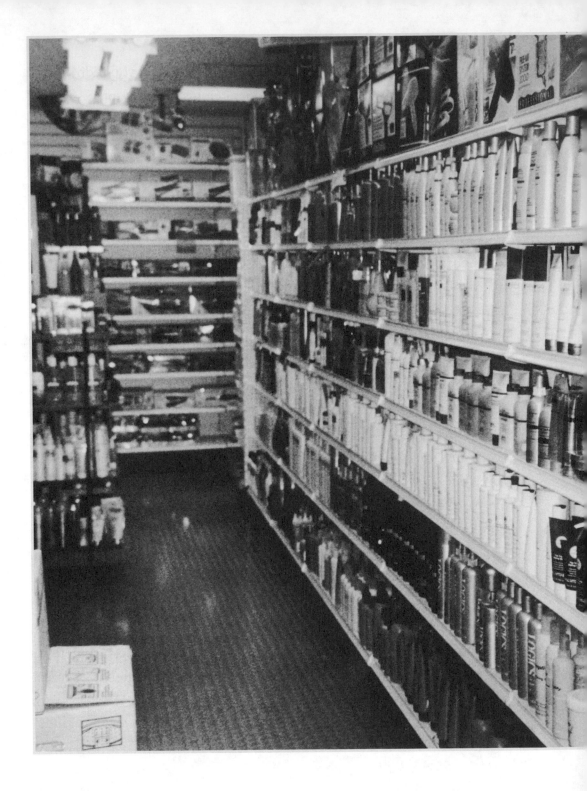

What's in a Name?

Focusing on the basics seems simple and straightforward enough until we look at the hundreds of products making competing claims on your hair and pocketbook. When it comes to the question of what's best to use, I can't and won't avoid the issue of cost. Some of the best products available are comparatively expensive, and some are quite cheap. As for weighing in on the debate over higher-priced brand names versus less-expensive ones, my approach is to merely explain to you the types of products to use for your hair. I don't want to confuse you with brand names; there are so many it can be overwhelming. Plus, new-and-improved products are launched by the cosmetic companies every year. If you know what type you need, then you'll be able to wisely pick and choose products that will work best for your hair. When it comes to expensive brand names versus tried-and-true brands, my bottom line is that the choice is yours. I'm just here to share with you some possibilities, so that you can make an intelligent choice.

A good stylist's priority is your hair, not the product. If your stylist is honest with you, he may recommend a mix-and-match approach to purchasing hair-care products. Don't get me wrong: The best product lines pride themselves on their quality, whether it's the shampoo, conditioner, or what have you. But let's face it, after you've paid $20 for shampoo, your pocketbook may need a break. There's nothing wrong with using shampoo X with conditioner Y, as long as the products themselves have proven they can do the job. I'm well aware that people do develop product loyalty, and that's fine. However, I think it's important to focus on hair-care ABC's. As you'll see when you read further, understanding your hair well is what leads a smart woman to use the best available products.

Know Thyself

Experimentation—and yes, some of this will be old-fashioned trial and error—in choosing the right hair-care products can be helped by employing the knowledge you've accumulated from learning some basic facts about hair and being real about how you live your life. Given your lifestyle and your hair type and texture, you can make some intelligent decisions. That doesn't solve the problem of knowing if a product actually works for you; the only way to know that is to use it. Be prepared to spend some money as you try out different shampoos, conditioners, lotions, and gels, but, no matter what it costs, no matter whose name is on it, if it doesn't work for you, it doesn't work.

Again, the simplest way to shuffle through all those products and find what works is to recognize your texture and realize what your specific hair texture requires versus that of straight hair. Curly, kinky, wavy hair, whether it's coarse, medium, or fine textured, long or short, is naturally drier than straight hair. That simply means that at any given time, the amount of moisture contained in curly hair (with kinky hair being at the end of the continuum) is less than that in straight hair. It's also more difficult for the sebum that the scalp's oil glands provide to reach the entire hair shaft of someone with curly or kinky hair than someone with straight hair. (Let's call it a hair geometry postulate: the shortest distance between two points is a straight hair!)

Remember the cuticle? Straight hair has smooth, flat cuticles while curly hair has raised, open cuticles, making it susceptible to much more dryness and frizz. That word *frizz* is often used derisively when describing curly and kinky hair. I'm on a mission to delete it from your vocabulary! All day long I hear my curly-locked clients complain that their hair is frizzy. Well, all curly hair is frizzy, particularly the hair close to the hairline. Frizziness is a function of your hair's having multiple textures, or its reaction to your body's heat—in other words, it is part of the hair's texture, not a mortal sin. I believe that extremely kinky hair gets a bad rap not because of its inherent curliness, but because it often becomes even drier from the products and treatments some of you have been using and overusing.

No single product (or product line, for that matter) can be all things to all heads. Finding the right hair-care products for you, even when using sound guidelines, still requires some investigation. But once you know what it is you need, a world of beauty supply opens up.

Shampoos

Myth: Many women have been raised to believe that hair should be shampooed frequently.

The good news is that there are many more products available than ever before to work with curly, kinky, and so-called frizzy hair. Let's start with shampoos. Shampoo is probably the most overrated product on the market, particularly for nonstraight hair. First, and this may come as a big surprise to you, dear reader, shampoo is for the scalp, not the hair; conditioners are for the hair, not the scalp. As I mentioned before, your scalp produces oil to moisturize and give luster to the hair. The scalp, as the "manufacturing site," is what gets truly dirty. (If you've ever walked through the streets of a hot, humid, heavily polluted city and bathed afterward, you know what I mean.) And were it not for your hair, you could use your favorite body cleanser on your head. Why? Because whatever works to clean the rest of your skin would be just fine, a fact that bald-headed folks learned a long time ago. When you shampoo your hair, you're removing vital oils from it and drying it out. It's your scalp that you should be shampooing and your hair that you should be protecting.

Shampoo is pH balanced so that it won't wreck your hair. But shampoo will promote big, frizzy, dry, dull hair if not used properly. Nevertheless, I'm sure you've heard numerous shampoo ads touting the importance of pH balance as if that alone were the secret ingredient for fabulous, fuller, and hands-down-healthier hair. Marketers know what they're doing, but the down and dirty of it is that shampoo was, is, and always will be for cleaning your scalp. It's just formulated in such a way as not to ruin your hair in the process. All that I'm really saying is that choosing a shampoo for many of you is about finding a gentle, effective scalp cleanser that doesn't unduly affect your hair by drying it out or leaving a residue.

You can overshampoo your hair regardless of what texture it is, i.e., whether your hair is fine or thick. Remember, it's your scalp you should be shampooing. Washing and scrubbing the hair itself dries your hair out. I can understand the temptation to vigorously scrub your hair if you're using products that have a wax base, such as pomades, greases, or other products that build up on the hair. They make the hair dull, and attract dust. If I could get you to wean yourself of those kinds of products and instead switch to water-soluble styling products, I'd be happier.

You actually can clean your hair a smart way by rinsing rather than shampooing it. If you like, you can even rinse hair six times a day. There's no harm done, and it does some good if this gets you to condition your hair every time you rinse. This way you can get your hair as clean as you need to without putting shampoo on it.

Remember when you had a pimple, back in the day, and they told you alcohol would make it go away? But what swabbing the pimple with alcohol really did was overactivate the oil gland, causing it to produce more oil, which, ta da! made an even bigger pimple. The same concept holds true with shampooing oily hair. Each time you shampoo, the oil glands go into overtime and that results in oily, flat hair with dry ends. You end up with just the opposite of what you wanted. Talk about a vicious cycle!

The shampoo you choose should be based on low detergent content and how the hair feels immediately after shampooing (and before applying conditioner). Having the hair squeaky clean is not necessarily the best objective. It can mean that too much oil has been stripped away. This often happens when you use a shampoo with a high detergent content. If your hair (and scalp) have a lot of waxy buildup, it might be reasonable to alternate shampoos. Shampoos vary in the amount of detergent they contain. If you want to continue to use a high-detergent shampoo such as a clarifying shampoo, I recommend that it be used sparingly—once a month, or once every two months, depending on how naturally dry your hair is, just to remove any buildup. During other washings, use a milder shampoo.

Given the importance of hydration to all woman with kinky, curly, or wavy hair, you would be smart to shop for shampoos and conditioners that are formulated for dry hair, or for chemically treated hair. Or, regardless of how you defined yourself on the last census, try some of those shampoos and conditioners specifically designed for African-American women, since the good ones are formulated for drier, more vulnerable hair.

Look for shampoos that contain the least amount of man-made chemicals and instead list naturally derived ingredients. A few ingredients you should learn to recognize are the following:

Sodium laureth sulfate is a mild cleansing agent derived from coconut oil. It's excellent for its foaming and cleaning properties and gentle on both hair and scalp.

Lauramide DEA is the principal fatty acid in coconut oil. This fatty acid is used as a softener and foaming agent.

Propylene glycol, which is also from coconut oil extract, helps the hair retain moisture.

Cocamidopropyl betaine is the same as coconut oil sodium chloride, or coconut oil salt, and is used as an astringent. (Astringents have antibacterial properties and are used in scalp cleansers.)

Ammonium lauryl sulfate is a mild acidic surfactant that ammonium salt comes from.

All products, even those containing naturally derived substances, will have some preservatives to prevent bacterial growth and contamination.

(There's no getting around that, nor would you want to.) A widely used preservative such as *methylparaben* has antimicrobial properties that can cause allergic reactions. No matter what you use, remember that when shampooing, you should concentrate on the scalp.

Finally, a few words regarding dandruff shampoos: Please don't use them! Dandruff shampoos contain ingredients such as tar or selenium disulfide, which dry out the scalp and hair, causing your oil glands to overreact. (Remember my example of the alcoholic pimple?) There are effective ways to manage mild cases of dandruff without stripping your scalp and hair of oil. (For severe, persistent dandruff, you should be treated by a dermatologist.) For many of you, I know there's not much choice. Some kind of dandruff-controlling shampoo (or those formulated to treat *seborrhea* or *psoriasis*) is necessary for your hair care and self-esteem. If that's the case, use the dandruff shampoo in conjunction with a conditioner and a monthly deep-conditioning treatment. Later on in this chapter I'll introduce you to a delicious choice of essential oils and some herbal remedies that can help soothe and repair your scalp in the meantime.

Conditioners

Myth: Conditioner makes hair limp and flat.

Hair conditioners work like lotions for the hair. They moisturize the hair, helping to do what sebum oil from the oil glands does naturally. In addition to their moisturizing function, conditioners make it easier to comb through hair when it's wet so that you don't rip through the hair and break it. A good conditioner can do many things for your hair, but conditioners do not "repair" damaged hair, so don't believe that hype. However, they certainly are a necessity in any healthy hair regimen.

If you have kinky or curly hair, there is no such thing as overconditioning. After every shampoo, follow up with a nice conditioner on the ends. Regardless of your hair type, the necessity of conditioning your hair is especially true for you women with nonstraight hair. Yet, if it's so important, why is it that I'm telling you to apply the conditioner just to the ends? The truth of the matter is that the hair that is closest to your scalp gets the benefit of any sebum coming from your oil glands. So, it will already be provided with its own conditioner. It is the ends, the hair farthest away from the scalp, that most need and will benefit from conditioner. Remember, kinky hair is naturally drier because the oil doesn't get to the "end of the line."

How you rinse the conditioner is most important. Distribute your conditioner throughout your hair. (Those of you with volume needn't fear conditioner like straight-haired women do. Their concern is that the conditioner will weigh down the hair, making it limp. You, on the other hand, have a lot of fragile strands that are incompletely moisturized by sebum. They'll love you for lavishing on conditioner!) The art of using conditioner is that you should rinse it out just enough to leave your hair feeling soft. Learning what "soft" is for your hair will take some practice. This is an example of the kind of experimentation you'll need to do as you get more intimate with your hair. Let's say, for instance, after rinsing the conditioner out your hair feels squeaky clean. If that's the case, then you've rinsed too much.

If you wear your hair naturally kinky or curly, the best curl is obtained as you're rinsing your conditioner out. That's true whether you've just cleaned your hair by shampooing or water-rinsing. Hair should always be dripping wet and soft after you rinse out your conditioner. Maintaining that softness during conditioning is best achieved by deep conditioning under a portable hood dryer, wearing a plastic cap. Yes, I said a hood dryer! Make no mistake, a hood dryer is your hair's best friend. It serves many a purpose for your hair, from caring to styling. It's best to condition with heat after every shampooing, be that once a week, twice a week, or once every two weeks.

Protein conditioners are a must-have for many women who chemically alter their hair. The protein in the conditioners is the same as the protein that makes up your hair: *keratin*. These conditioners are usually used in conjunction with a heat or steam application. During that process the protein passes through your cuticle to get to the cortex, strengthening the hair shaft and increasing its elasticity.

As great as they are, if used too often, products with a high percentage of protein can dry out your hair. For those of you who can use protein conditioners, I recommend that you alternate them with a moisture pack, which is an everyday conditioner containing some protein, or a moisturizing conditioner.

Cream rinses are strictly for very fine hair. They make it easy to comb, but generally don't do much else, so while they may be marketed as conditioners, they really aren't.

Leave-in conditioner is for hair that needs that extra softening. Mineral oil is an ingredient of leave-in conditioner. I often use a leave-in conditioner if I'm going to use styling lotion or gel to create a natural-looking style. Leave-in conditioner prevents the hair from becoming hard or stiff.

The cosmetic companies now have a few high-end products that have taken advantage of the popularity of moisturizing hair treatments.

For instance, there are preshampoo conditioning treatments that can run you about $30. Instead, I'd recommend that you get an inexpensive conditioner like *cholesterol,* which, while serious as a heart attack, won't give you one because of the price! This humble, inexpensive product has been around for years. Cholesterol is a heavy, thick conditioner that can be used two ways: one method is as a preshampoo treatment to protect extremely dry hair prior to shampooing; or, after shampooing, cholesterol can be applied to the hair, and then you spend ten to fifteen minutes under the dryer as the cholesterol works to soften and moisturize the shaft. After a cholesterol pretreatment, proceed with a moisturizing shampoo on the scalp, rinse well, and condition as you normally would.

Lanolin, derived from the oil glands of sheep, is intended to help the skin absorb and hold moisture. It's used as an ingredient in products such as lotions and conditioners.

Castor oil has been used as a cosmetic since antiquity. (It's been found in ancient Egyptian tombs.) Although many of us recall its use as a laxative, when it's applied to hair it's a moisturizer. Castor oil is used on kinky hair, which tends to be spongy, and is great on frizzy, coarse hair.

Castor oil is another great product for preshampoo treatments. As a pretreatment, apply the oil to your hair and then sit under the hood dryer for approximately ten to fifteen minutes. The oil softens coarse hair. When done under the dryer, shampoo your hair to remove the oil and recondition with a moisturizing conditioner or your normal conditioner.

Castor oil has one more important use, as far as hair is concerned. Because it is rich in essential fatty acids, it's often used as an emulsifier. (Emulsifiers are what makes it possible for certain liquids to have a creamy consistency, as opposed to separating in the bottle like oil and water do.) Therefore, emulsifiers are found in grooming products like hair creams and lotions.

Another product that has a function similar to castor oil is a versatile oil (or fat) called *shea butter,* derived from a tree common to West and Central Africa. It protects and coats the skin and hair. The shielding quality of shea butter makes it an effective barrier to the sun's ultraviolet rays, which can dry your hair.

Essential Oils

As you may have guessed, I am an advocate of using nontoxic natural products whenever possible. Certain commonly practiced treatments, even though they use natural products, may not be beneficial or may even be harmful to your hair. One such culprit is the popular hot oil treatment. Hot oil treatments are marketed as if they add oil and moisture to your hair. (Hot oil treatments are right up there with clay masks as being mandatory for serious beauty queens!) Many women do the treatments thinking they are treating their dry hair. That is a big misconception. Oil removes oil by breaking it down so that it can be washed out of the hair. A hot oil treatment is counterproductive if your ultimate purpose is to add more oil to your hair. The treatments are best used to remove buildup on your hair and scalp, and they are particularly good for gently removing color buildup from temporary and semipermanent hair color.

A more sensible treatment for a dry scalp would be to use natural essential oils massaged into the scalp. Oils work wonders in normalizing the scalp by restoring essential oils to it. By itself, massaging opens product-clogged pores and reinvigorates a scalp dried from poor circulation, or from—you guessed it!—overshampooing. The combination of massage and an essential oil gives you a simultaneous moisturizing and restorative treatment.

There are many great oils for the scalp. The ones I'd like to introduce you to are those I've come to discover through the very trial-and-error process I invited you to do. I started to make the conversion to lightweight essential oils because I found too many women of color, and others with nonstraight hair, still using wax-based oils and pomades. I can understand the attachment to these products. They are the stuff of folk legend. But ladies, the science of hair care has advanced into the twenty-first century. Why don't you join us here? Using these lightweight oils serves you far better. They permit all of you with kinky or frizzy hair to still add luster and shine, while fortifying your scalp and hair. Additionally, some of the oils have astringent or antibacterial properties. Here are some of my favorites:

Tea tree oil is a soothing, healing astringent that works by stimulating the scalp as it disinfects.

Comfrey is a powerful healing herb. As an agent, it can aid in destroying bacteria and healing cuts, abrasions, and chemical burns from relaxers or coloring. Comfrey oil contains a natural hormone called *allantoin,* known for its bone-strengthening and skin cell–restorative properties. Allantoin also serves as a natural retardant for hair loss.

Eucalyptus oil has significant antiseptic and antibacterial qualities. Its active germicidal agent prevents infection, and it leaves your scalp feeling cool, tingly, and soothed.

Although not an oil per se, *witch hazel,* a tree bark distillate, is used as a cleansing astringent that leaves behind volatile oils and amino acids, which condition and stimulate the scalp.

Almond oil is a wonderful moisturizer and scalp soother. Not only does it contain protein and other important minerals for the hair, but it acts like your own sebum, encouraging moisture retention.

Jojoba oil is the gold standard of essential oils, thanks to its many properties. Jojoba is rich in nutrients that protect, restore, and moisturize your hair. Often hot oil treatments and conditioners contain jojoba oil because it aids in the treatment of hair problems stemming from extreme dryness.

The Finishing Touches

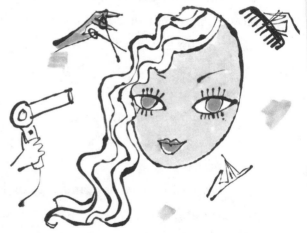

Now that you've washed, conditioned, and are on the verge of styling your hair, it's time we moved on to the finishing touches. I know your ideal is to have your hair look its best, feel soft, and practically invite people to touch it. While it would be great to find the one product that will condition and style your hair, the fact is, your hair texture and the end result (your vision or ideal) will help determine what you'll need. For some of you it may turn out to be one product. For others, a combination of products is best. Understanding the categories of styling products is essential to making the right choices.

Let's begin with *silicone* (sometimes called silicone serum) and anti-frizz products containing *dimethicone,* a silicone-based product. Silicone is a water-soluble liquid with a clear, viscous consistency. You can use the liquid in either spray or squeeze applications. Despite its oily feel, silicone won't make the hair oily and is great for forming curls and/or blow-drying hair straight because it smooths out the cuticle. If you're trying to combat frizzy hair, then when your hair is wet, that is, at its most "frizz-less," apply your product.

Great as it is as a styling product, silicone is a plastic. This means that over time silicone can build up on your hair and dry it out. Because of that, it should be used on top of a light leave-in conditioner. All silicone products, whether for curly styles or straight looks, should be applied to wet hair. After gently squeezing out the water, the hair should be either blown dry or air dried. Don't towel-dry your hair; the towel causes you to rough up the cuticle, leaving you with frizzy hair (again). Also, if you towel-dry your hair, the silicone sits on top of it, making it feel and look sticky and greasy.

Sculpting lotions are great for curly hair when coupled with a leave-in conditioner. They have a slight, crisp hold that can be broken up after your hair is dry.

Gels stiffen the hair and are for hard-to-hold styles that offer little movement. A gel's consistency is thick, which is good for short hairstyles. However, I need to caution you that regular gels dry hard, and combing through the hair after applying gel may cause your hair to break. There is such a thing as a *conditioning gel*. Like the name implies, this kind of gel isn't as hard on the hair. It doesn't dry hard, even though it holds a curl. You'll notice the difference when you apply conditioning gel: The hair doesn't feel crunchy or hard, but instead feels soft and firm.

Pomades are used to calm stray hairs, and add luster and movement to stiff hair. Pomades tend to be wax-based and can coat the hair, so proceed with caution. (Ask the old folks what they used to say about Brylcreem: "A little dab'll do ya.")

Setting lotion is a lightweight liquid version of sculpting lotion. It's perfect to use with wet sets and while you're blow-drying. Setting lotion adheres to almost any hair type without drying hard or leaving a sticky residue, and adds shine and body. If you have chemically straightened hair, setting lotion is an ideal styling product for you.

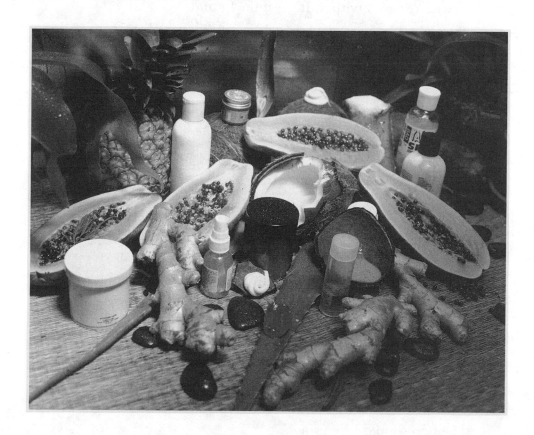

Questions & Answers

Q: The more humid it gets, the frizzier my hair gets, especially after I wash it. What can I do?

A: Humidity just loves dry hair. Humidity is nothing more than atmospheric moisture, and the drier your hair is, the more humidity wreaks havoc with it. It's as if the humidity coming in contact with a dry surface, your hair, is saying, "I'll be all over you like white on rice." Try shampooing less and conditioning more to fill in the cracked, dry cuticle that causes frizzy hair.

Q: I have fine hair and I can't seem to find a product that doesn't feel sticky on my hair. Any suggestions?

A: Make sure whatever styling lotion you buy has a lightweight consistency. If it is lightweight, you can use more of it than you would a heavier product. The rule of thumb is that you apply it to your wet hair (when it's not frizzy). I really mean wet hair, not towel dried. Otherwise, anything that you apply to your hair after towel-drying will feel sticky.

Q: After I shampoo my hair, it gets big and frizzy. What kind of shampoo should I be using?

A: All shampoo contains some amount of detergent, which will dry your hair. That's just as true for shampoos that are formulated for moisturizing dry hair. If your hair is already dry, and you've shampooed it (as opposed to water-rinsing the hair), you need to make it a practice to follow every shampooing with a deep conditioner, and then a lightweight leave-in conditioner. Feel free to be generous with conditioner, and try using shampoos for chemically treated hair. They work well for curly, dry hair.

Q: I have fine, curly hair. Conditioner usually makes my hair flat. What do I do?

A: Just because you have fine hair doesn't mean you should do without conditioner, right? The best way for you to use it is to apply your conditioner only to your ends, not near the scalp, which will make your hair flat. Perhaps (and you can experiment with this) you could apply some conditioner around your hairline if it tends to get frizzy. For you, a little bit of conditioner will go a long way.

Q: I have a kinky-type natural cut, and my scalp is dry. What do I do?

A: I'm beginning to sound like the proverbial broken record: Apply your conditioner sparingly, making sure it winds up in your hair, not on your scalp. After conditioning, massage a lightweight essential oil, like almond oil, into your scalp.

Q: I recently bought a new conditioner that everyone is swearing by for my thick, curly hair. I paid $18 for it and it does work, but after I use it once or twice, it's practically all gone. I just can't afford $18 every two weeks. Do you have any suggestions?

A: Shop around for conditioners that are half the price, and buy two of them. Spend the money on experimenting with less expensive products and I bet you'll find one that goes farther than your pocketbook does!

Q: I would love to get my hair done by a stylist, but my budget won't allow me to be anything but a do-it-myselfer. What should I do?

A: Money is a reality, and I respect that. Save yours up, all the while getting some free word-of-mouth about whom you might like to go to. It's the best way to find the right person for you. Once you've settled on the stylist, get your money's worth by asking as many questions as you can so that you can learn as much as possible about how to care for your hair.

In the meantime, here's a suggestion for financing your appointment: Start telling your friends and family *right now* that instead of gifts such as clothing, jewelry, and so on, a gift certificate or a contribution toward a gift certificate at your favorite salon would be much appreciated and used. Depending on how many folks love you, in no time you should have enough to have your hair professionally treated, conditioned, or colored at least twice a year. When they see what it does for your looks, who knows? Maybe your favorite aunt will spring for more frequent visits!

In all seriousness, try to save up for at least one treatment by a professional. You'll be delighted at how much you can learn about your own hair, good products, and some tips about care and styling. One visit may inspire you to take even better care of your hair. So, while you may not be able to afford to go to the stylist as often as you'd like, you can strive to use the best products and the most sensible care. That kind of inspiration is priceless.

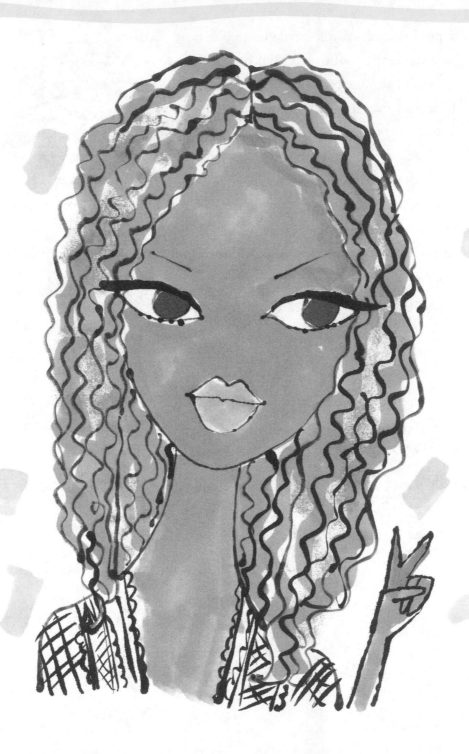

Chapter 3

It's Your Thing!
Do What You Want to Do!

Your God-given Glory

The American hair market (which is pitched largely to straight- or wavy-haired Caucasians) has not been specific enough about how women in the entire spectrum of curly hair should care for their tresses. As a result, women with kinky hair (primarily, but not exclusively, women of African, Jewish, or Latin descent) and women with curly hair have been confused (to put it mildly) about where they belong in the hair-care continuum.

To all of you women with moderately curly to extremely curly hair, I'll tell you this right now: Your hair-care regimen should be closer to that of women with kinky hair than it is to that of women with silky-straight hair. And that's why this chapter is devoted to the natural hair of all women with "ethnic" hair types—in other words, to those of you who have bowed down to your original texture and given the chemicals a break. Yeah, girl, I'm talkin' to you!

Let's imagine that at some point in a woman's life she decides to or has to wear her hair natural. Some women voluntarily return their hair to its God-given state for aesthetic reasons, and some do it because of health reasons, to give overprocessed hair and a damaged scalp time to grow or heal. Whatever the reason or reasons, I want you to know how to make what you were born with look good. How you care for it will lead you to a better understanding of which approaches to use to maintain its natural beauty.

Many women today are coming to a more holistic way of living. Your spiritual selves have taken a front-row seat in how you live your lives. There's a greater emphasis on what you eat, what you put on your bodies, and whether you get sufficient exercise. Also, more and more women are subscribing to a homeopathic approach to their health, with wellness of mind and body being the ultimate goal.

For some women, an examination of how they live has led them to question contemporary society's dependence on altered food, and altered appearance in order to be considered desirable. This may mean eating only organically produced foods, or it may mean a decision not to alter their hair's texture. Natural hair, then, whether it's short or long, in a 'fro, curls, or locks, is an emphatic declaration of who they are.

Myth: Kinky hair is durable, strong, and coarse. You can use whatever products and processes you like on it, and the hair will be just fine.

What has become clear and shocking to me when consulting with clients—no matter what they want, what they have, or where they've come from—is the lack of knowledge about their hair's original, natural texture. Being one of the few hairstylists who specializes in all textures, what I have found to be true is that many women with gorgeous curly and kinky hair often don't learn how to truly care for what they possess.

Glorifying your hair texture and knowing how to maintain it is a first step. It is the beginning of an honest approach to wearing and caring for your crowning glory. So, starting from this point on I'll be sharing maintenance techniques and alternative styling methods. By the time we're done, you will have gotten to know how to make what you have look good, just like it was meant to. Learning what makes natural hair look good (and stay healthy) is just as important for women with processed hair as it is for other women. Some women have scarcely acknowledged the type of hair they were born with because they don't truly care about their hair in its natural state. They know it's curly, or they know it's coiled and kinky, but that's about it.

In a perfect world, the texture of one's hair should be of little or no concern when it comes to self-esteem. But, given our history, most women of ethnic origin who wear their curly or kinky hair in its natural state wouldn't be caught dead without a perm or a hot-comb press. There are still a few sisters who struggle with what we call "hair hatred." Hair hatred stems from the belief that silky-straight hair is inherently superior to coiled hair, and from never being told how to wear and truly care for kinky hair.

Some of them come to me and announce that their hair is nappy or frizzy, so can we just relax it, please? Or "Can we just blow-dry it straight?" they anxiously ask me. "Because I hate my hair." Well, misery does have company. My work has introduced me to many a Jewish or Hispanic woman who despises her naturally curly or kinky and dark tresses.

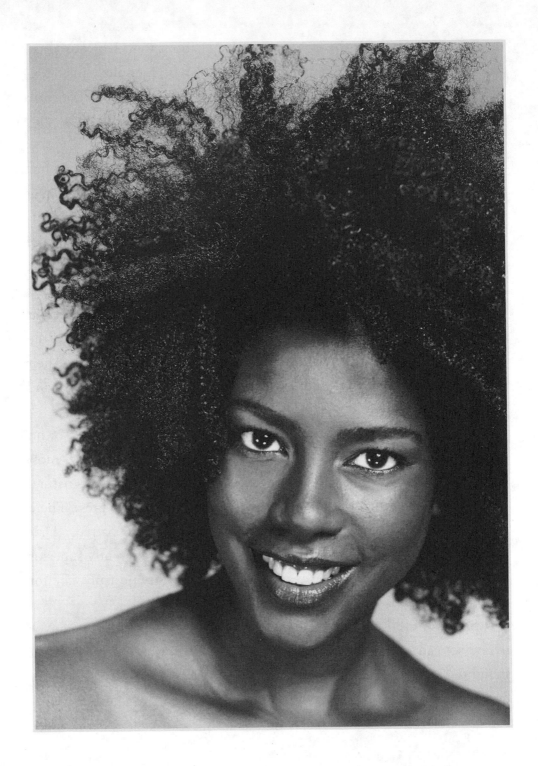

And why? Because they have never been shown how to make their hair, with its particular texture, look good.

It's time for all that foolishness to stop! It's time you considered a holistic approach to the care and maintenance of unprocessed hair. Once again we'll start with the basics: shampooing and conditioning.

Basic Training

For unprocessed hair, the use of products is minimized, because protecting the hair from chemicals isn't necessary. However, the basics in terms of cleaning and conditioning are very much the same. Let's begin with those. For starters, shampoo less. The hair as it exists naturally is dry to begin with. If you've gone and, for whatever reasons (and I hope your reasons are legit), chemically treated your hair in the past, you have further dried it. How you shampoo and condition your vulnerable hair will be the deciding factors in maintaining its health, and making it possible for you to have the freedom to choose even more styling options in the future.

Shampooing

You can overshampoo your hair regardless of what texture it is, or whether your hair is fine or thick. There are those of you who feel like your hair gets dirty or oily so fast that you've gotten into the habit of shampooing every day. When you do that, you're stripping your hair of its much needed sebum. There really is an alternative to daily shampooing: As I stated earlier, simply rinse it.

When you feel the need or the necessity for cleaning and styling, just rinse your hair with plenty of hot water, all the while massaging your scalp with your finger pads to stimulate the flow of blood. At the same time that you're encouraging blood flow, you're dislodging sediment and residue, but not stripping away sebum. I can't stress enough the importance of keeping hygienically clean hair and unclogged pores (which is why I discourage my clients from using wax-based products), and rinsing the hair, essentially cleaning it often enough so that it's never funky.

It's all in the hands. The trick is to rinse until it *feels* clean to your touch. When you've arrived at that point (or when everyone else is banging on the bathroom door) then you're ready for conditioning.

Conditioning

For naturally drier, kinky hair there is no such thing as overconditioning. Conditioning your hair is truly a sensual experience. You should massage your conditioner throughout the hair after first applying it to the ends, where it is most needed. Whether you've just shampooed or rinsed, how you rinse out the conditioner is most important. With your fingers, massage and comb through your conditioner-laden hair and feel it move. Swing it, running your hands over it back and forth. Feel your curl separate and clump together in tangle-free locks. I promise you, this will be a luxurious and intimate experience just between you and your hair. It will teach you to get to know your hair at its most desirable texture—a soft curl pattern with no frizz. Now, remember, this is how you want it to look and feel when it's dry.

The art of using conditioner is that you should rinse it out just enough to leave your hair feeling soft. As I explained in Chapter 2, recognizing what "soft" is for your hair will take some practice. As you become sensitive to your hair's texture, you'll know whether what your fingertips are feeling is a thin coating of conditioner or just wet hair.

Let's return to conditioning and rinsing. If your intention is to wear your hair naturally curly or kinky, the best way to have your curl look beautiful will be determined when you're rinsing out your conditioner. Whether you've just shampooed or water-rinsed, how you handle your hair as you rinse out the conditioner is very important. It's what I consider the first step in styling natural hair.

Have It Your Curly, Kinky Way!

Hair should always be dripping wet and soft after you rinse out your conditioner. Now is the time to shake or squeeze the water out and apply your leave-in conditioner and/or conditioning gel. Maintaining that softness after conditioning is best achieved by drying the hair under a portable hood dryer with a plastic cap. It's best to condition under a dryer after every shampoo, be that once a week or twice a week. Now you're ready to go on.

If you have curly hair, how you apply product is the next important step in keeping your hair as close as possible to that undisturbed, flawless curl you discovered while washing it. Apply product as you did with your erotic, intimate conditioning rinse, that is, evenly, with an open hand. Do not run your fingers through your hair, upsetting the curl. Instead, section your hair and gently squeeze in leave-in conditioner and/or conditioning gel.

For women with kinky hair, castor oil can be used as a preshampoo treatment. One of the advantages of kinky hair is its sponginess, which means that it can "drink up" a substance like castor oil. Because of that, you don't have to worry that applying castor oil will weigh down your hair.

If your hair is long and thick, find your style when your hair is wet, not towel dried, and apply your product then. Your hair is so much more pliable when it's wet, and that's when you can really set the curl—by twisting or braiding your hair. Back in the day, women worked on their hair in sections by braiding or twisting parts of their hair that they wanted to get out of the way in preparation for pressing it. One of the marvelous things (although many didn't think so at the time) that came out of that practice was the beautiful, sculpturelike shapes that were liberated as the braids or twists were undone. Twisting and braiding are now recognized as styling options that texturize your hair without chemicals. Just like the wet set and thermal pressing, they are temporary, yet they offer you the versatility of an elegant or funky hairstyle, depending on your mood and taste.

That's the key: Twist it, braid it, have it your way! All you have to do is start with your wet, conditioned hair. On cool mornings, use a hood dryer on your hair, but during warm weather, letting your hair air-dry is just fine. Or you can use a diffuser, an attachment to your blow-dryer that simulates the effect of a hood dryer. It allows you, as you are drying your hair, more mobility so that you can concentrate on, or spot-dry, sections of hair to add more volume.

One last tip for keeping your glorious natural hair beautiful: If you can afford it, I advise using satin pillowcases, or, if that's too out there, a satin scarf as opposed to a cotton one on your head when you sleep. Cotton fibers can absorb oil and have just enough roughness to tangle your hair and cause it to mat. Satin will help keep your curl undisturbed, and your hair will slide across the fabric without frizzing.

Knowledge Is Power

Now that you've spent some time learning about the beauties of natural kinky hair, even if wearing it natural is not your thing, you'll appreciate why it is the preferred choice of many other women. Whatever your personal style, I think it's good for you to know how to care for your hair in its natural state. Armed with knowledge of (and, I hope, more appreciation for) your natural hair, you may just decide one day to change your style. If that day comes, you won't have any fear of taking care of your crowning glory.

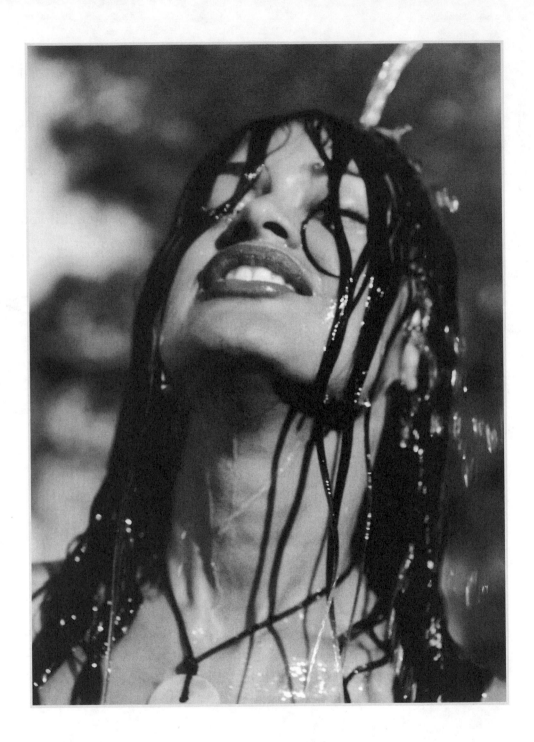

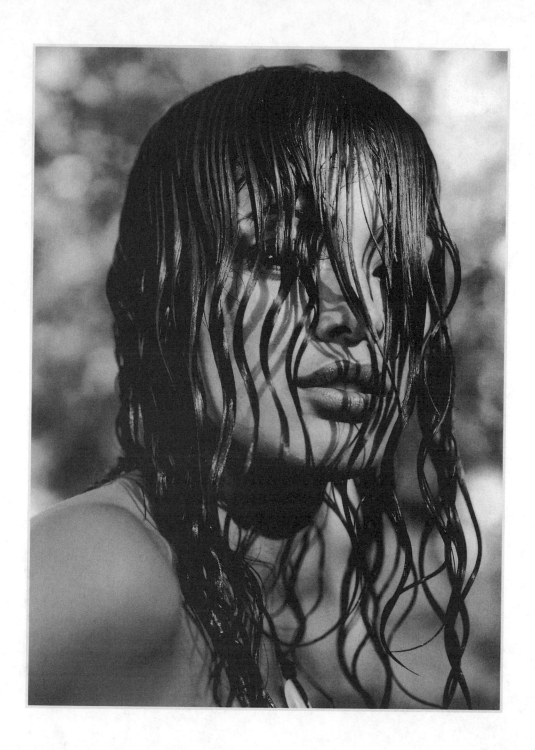

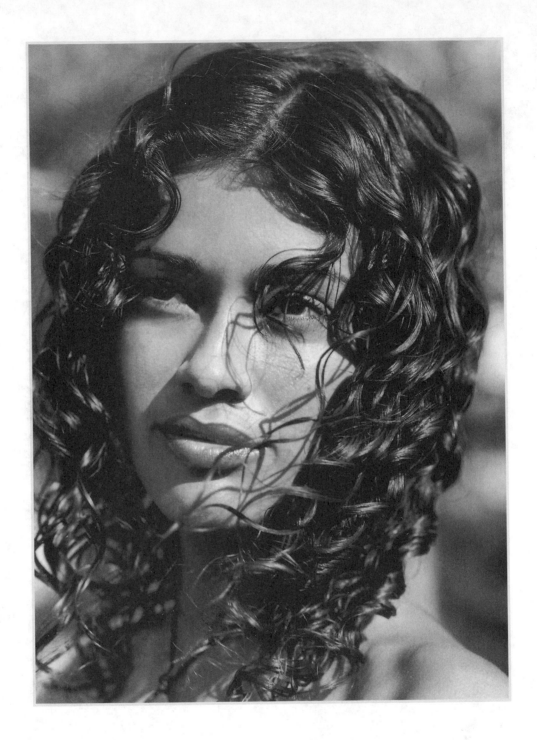

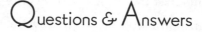

Questions & Answers

Q: I wear my hair natural. How often do I need to get it cut or trimmed?

A: Cutting, of course, depends on the length that you want to maintain. But as for trimming, I want to illustrate a point by talking about two heads of hair, one coarse and one fine. Even though a fine head of hair may be described as a thick head of hair, meaning lots of fine hairs per square inch, when it comes to routine maintenance needs, the thick but fine hair needs to be trimmed more frequently. Why? Because the ends of fine hair are more apt to split than those of coarser hair. Fine hair, no matter how thick it is, is a different and more fragile grade than coarse hair.

When it's time to get your hair cut, I don't recommend thinning the hair or razor cutting. The best stylists will cut your hair with a scissors and comb.

Q: I have soft, kinky natural hair that I'd like to grow longer. How often should I have it cut?

A: I advise that you get your hair cut every eight to ten weeks, depending on how coarse or fine your hair is. When you do get it cut, it's best that it be cut only after the hair's been blown out with a comb attachment. That way the stylist can more accurately see your hair's ends.

Q: My hair doesn't seem to grow past my chin and it's fine and fragile. Everyone else in my family has hair that grows like crazy. Am I doing something wrong?

A: If you were sitting in my chair the first question I'd ask is "How often do you get your hair cut?" I'd ask because a scalp full of fine hair is dramatically different from, for instance, a scalp full of coarse hair. Generally, fine hair is more fragile and needs to be cut or trimmed more often than coarse hair. So, it may indeed seem to be growing more slowly because the ends are splitting. You could well be gaining an inch at your root, but the hair that you've been hesitant to cut is probably popping off so much that you're losing an equivalent amount at your ends.

If it appears as though your hair is growing too slowly, or seems to have stopped growing, start getting it trimmed often, and treat it gently (using the appropriate shampoos, conditioners, and styling products) to avoid breaking it. I think you'll start to see a difference.

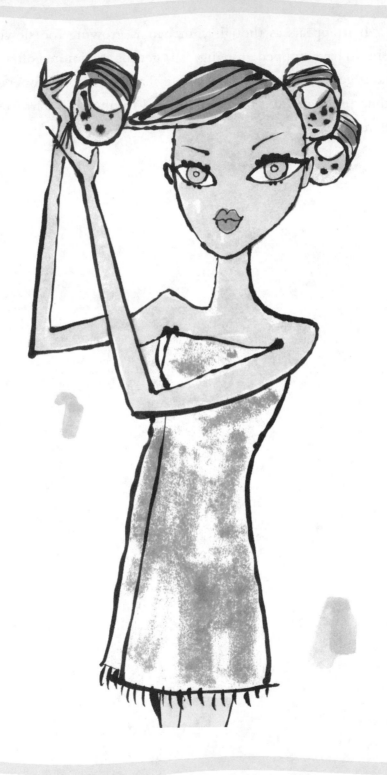

Chapter 4

Some Like It Wet

Your Grandmother Knows Something You Don't

The wet set is associated with little old ladies in their neighborhood salons. Thus, it takes the rap for not being trendy or hip because it requires that a woman spend her precious time under the dryer. Those old ladies may not be trendy, but there's one thing they are definitely better at, and that's maintaining healthy hair. They instinctively know that the wet set is a great method for styling hair that's been chemically relaxed. This chapter introduces you to the benefits of wet setting, including how to set your hair between salon visits, and shows you how to use various tools for some wonderful home styling.

The minute blow-dryers hit the market in the late sixties, the wet set started to go the way of sponge rollers. Who could argue with the convenience and ease of a blow-dryer? Who was going to think twice about what it took to get that special 'do every day in just a few minutes? Now you could go from dripping-wet-straight-out-of-the-shower to fabulous before the coffee finished brewing. Many of those blow-dryer fans have learned the hard way about the consequences of frequent blow-drying. By using them daily, convenient though they are, many women have sacrificed their hair. Don't be one of those. It ain't worth all that. You can actually maintain a great style, and your hair, by doing what your grandma did.

More often than not a client comes in and has one, two, three, or even more pictures of the same haircut on some model or celebrity. The hair is styled five different ways and my client can't figure out which one would best suit her. Or, after shuffling the pictures around she'll whisper to me: "She's so much younger, prettier, and skinnier than me!" All this before I can even comment on the hairstyle itself, because I rarely focus on anything but the hairstyle. (After all, I'm a hairstylist, not a plastic surgeon.) It's at this point that I get furious at all those "perfect" images that women think they have to live up to. The way I rebel against those images (after I've calmed myself down) and keep my own work exciting is to maintain my mind-set: There are no hard and fast rules about a woman's looks. It's not about which hairstyle you can or cannot wear; it's about maintaining healthy hair however you wear it.

Blow-Drying: Armed and Dangerous

Let's start with blow-drying. Before I get into the how's, I want you to repeat after me: Moderation is the key. Blow-drying offers vastly expanded options for women with nonstraight hair, allowing them to achieve certain looks right at home. However, this styling technique can be overdone so much that you can severely damage and dry out your hair. I tell my clients that blow-drying should be done only when necessary (and yes, I'll get to those of you who insist that necessity dictates that you blow-dry your hair every day). If done properly the results should last four to six days.

The curlier and coarser your hair is, the wetter your hair should be before you start to dry it. Using a nozzle on the end of your dryer will direct the heat exactly where you want it, while a natural-bristle brush stretches the sectioned hair smooth. If your hair is kinky, a blow-dryer with a comb attachment for pulling out the tightly wound coils is your appliance of choice. Just as I mentioned in Chapter 2, use a light leave-in conditioner before blow-drying so that the heat is burning off the conditioner and not your hair's natural oil.

Because of the demand for flawless-looking hair, appliances that professionals use, such as flat irons and curling irons, have become readily available to the general public. And guess what? Burned, broken hair is once again on the rise. Where a stylist may use these appliances on a client once a week, your average consumer gets hold of these very hot tools, some of which reach temperatures of 200° F, and uses, say, the flat iron every day. Then she calls the salon wanting to book an appointment for a deep conditioner. Well, there isn't any deep conditioner on the planet that's going to repair hair with little white scorched balls on the ends. Hair can't get more dead than that. Cut that stuff off. And stop ironing or curling your hair every day.

Always remember, your hair is a living thing (although the shaft itself has no nerve endings). When it isn't in the resting or shedding phase of its natural cycle, it is growing. For many of you who have overdone it with hot appliances, you can't tell that your hair is growing because your ends are minutely popping off. What happens is that you're constantly burning your ends, along with not having them cut on a regular basis. Even as you're gaining an inch at the roots, you're losing an inch on the ends, for a net gain (as they say in accounting) of zero growth. But to you, the "evidence" of no change in your hair's length morphs into the absolute conviction that your hair won't grow. Not to mention that you also complain that it's dry and you don't know why!

Humor me: Let's suppose your hair is chemically straightened, or that your natural color is brunette, but only you and your colorist know it. There you are walking around as blond as Pamela Anderson, blow-drying and ironing or curling your hair every day. What do you suppose might happen to hair like yours if you continue to heat it every day? I mean, come on now, even your Thanksgiving turkey has to come out of the oven sometime! I'm sorry. Am I being a little bit sarcastic? It's just that it's so distressing what some of you do to yourselves in the name of beauty. You'll have to forgive me, but I think you've got the picture: the one I need to show you of an attractive woman who's going to have one too many bad-hair days.

Look, the more natural the state of your hair, the more heat it can withstand. The less natural, the less heat. In other words, any prior process that you've applied to your hair, such as coloring and relaxing, weakens the shaft. That's why you should never, and I mean *never,* use stove or thermal irons on chemically straightened hair. And, if you want to use them on natural hair, I strongly advise that it be done by a professional. The direct heat is just too severe for the multiple textures on one's head. Instead, an electric iron is suggested as long as you follow the same precautions you would with blow-drying. Use the iron moderately, no more than once a week. Any more than that can be disastrous. Anything else you do may turn out to be "the straw that broke the camel's back." For those of you with relaxed hair, now that I've got you to at least think about putting down your gun, what, you ask, are you supposed to do? And that brings me to wet setting.

Girls Under the Hood

That trusty old hood dryer is still the best method of styling out there and the most versatile if you want a style that will last *and* keep your hair in good condition. It is the only styling option recommended for chemically straightened hair, whether you want full, voluminous, sleek, straight, or an evenly curly straw set. Hood dryers are also great for styling curly or kinky hair. There's no better way to set your own texture whether you roll it, twist it, pin it, or spiral it. The whole point is to set the hair when it is in its most unfrizzed, pliable state. Wet.

Wet setting your hair under a hood dryer takes longer than blow-drying; how long depends upon your hair's thickness. The wait is worth it because the set it gives you lasts longer than one obtained by blow-drying, plus the hair has more luster and shine, as there's no stress on the hair from a blow-dryer's intense heat. Come on, even you Type A's can park it once a week!

Another reason the wet set is so fabulous is that you're setting the hair when it's at its most pliable. Always make sure that your hair is saturated with water; don't towel-dry it. With wet, supple hair, it's easier to get it straight enough to roll or manipulate. Think about it: As you blow-dry, you are simultaneously pulling the hair straight as you dry it. If what you ultimately want is a style with some shape or curl, you have to then back up a step to curl the hair you just straightened. You don't have to do that when you wet set. You are essentially molding the style you want and then drying the hair so that the style is set.

The method by which you choose to style your hair can make or break (no pun intended) hair that has been chemically altered. If you are simply looking for an alternative to blow-drying because you have had it with the dry, brittle, broken, and limp hair that blow-drying can cause, roller setting your hair is a great choice. It is not only good for creating fabulous-looking styles, it's good for the hair itself. Roller setting is the safest, healthiest way to style your hair because the heat from a hood dryer is not a direct heat like that of a hot comb, flat iron, or curling iron. (As I said before, if your hair has been chemically straightened, don't even *think* about using irons on your hair.)

Roller setting is particularly beneficial for hair that is very fine and soft. Setting yourself up to make this process simple and habit forming is as important a step as any. Remember, I'm trying to get you to forgo the quick blow-drying you're used to. It's time you acquired those old-fashioned virtues of diligence and patience!

After shampooing and conditioning your hair, use a setting lotion or mousse while the hair is still very wet. Setting lotions have additional moisturizers and conditioners that give hair a bouncier, longer-lasting hold. Roller setting without a setting lotion, or at the very least a light leave-in conditioner, will dry out the ends of your hair. The next step uses the rollers. Simple plastic magnetic rollers will suffice. Avoid using sponge rollers because they'll break and dry the hair. Also, Velcro rollers are meant to be used strictly for dry sets, so they aren't suitable for a process that begins with wet hair.

Depending upon how you do it, you can achieve many styles regardless of your texture. In general, the roller size depends on the length of your hair and how tight a curl you want. For instance, you (or your stylist) can wrap your hair around huge rollers for straight styles. Very large rollers make almost no curl but provide body for those soft, straight, sleek styles with swing. (Say that three times fast!) When rolling, keep in mind that when wrapping your hair around the roller, less is more. Begin by

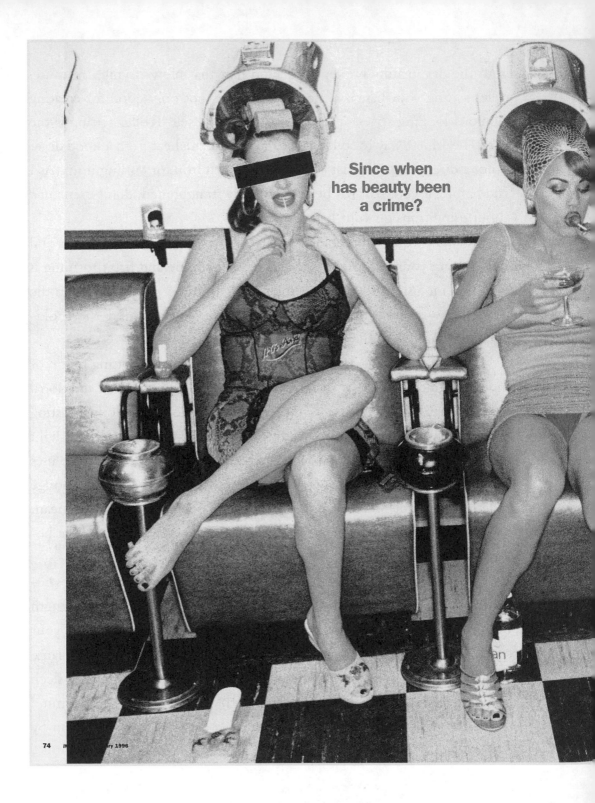

Since when has beauty been a crime?

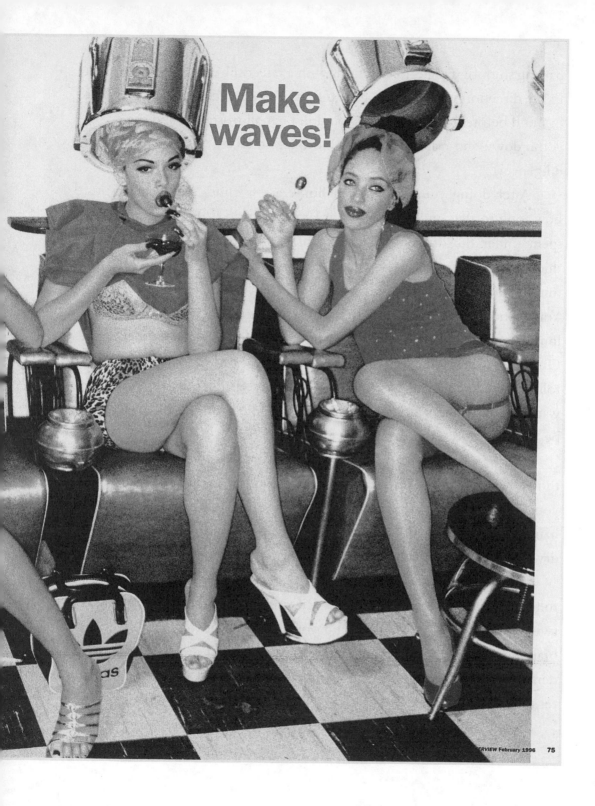

Make waves!

parting smooth, tangle-free sections with a tail comb and rolling your hair in the direction you want the hair to flow. You should have a desired style in mind before you start so that you don't get all frustrated and throw the comb down and reach for that ole blow-dryer. (Remember patience and diligence?)

After doing your own hair at home a few times, you'll know just how long to stay under the hood dryer. Each head is different, and time spent under the dryer will depend on your hair's length, texture, and thickness. Here's a technique to test for dryness: Let your hair cool for five minutes before you remove a roller from the longest part of your hair. You'll know that your hair is dry when it springs back firmly. If it falls limp, reroll it and resume drying until your "spring" test is successful. Once it's totally dry, let your hair cool for five minutes, take out the rollers, and brush your hair straight (if that's the intended style). If you want less body, blow-dry your hair with a paddle brush set on low. You'll be amazed at the shine and silkiness your hair has!

Another tip is that a roller set is the perfect hairstyling technique for those of you with relaxed hair who exercise. Before your workout, tie your hair back with a terry-cloth sweatband to absorb moisture at the hairline. After your workout, dry your hair from root to end with a blow-dryer that has a comb attachment on a warm to cool setting.

For those of you who are into funkier 'dos, you don't have to use rollers with your wet set. For instance, if you like a crimped look, you can twist your hair while it's wet, and you can make great wavy styles by braiding your hair. And to think that you can achieve these wild and wonderful looks without doing any damage to your hair! What could be better than that?

As I mentioned before, don't forget to sleep with a satin scarf or pillow cover because the satin will slide over the hair without absorbing your hair's oil. Cotton scarves and pillow covers absorb your hair's natural oil, causing it to dry out, mat, and tangle.

So, the sky's the limit, and the more you can do on your own, the more daring you'll become with a variety of styling options. Properly maintaining your hairstyle between salon visits, without the crutch of a hot appliance, is probably where you're most vulnerable. Don't be afraid to ask your stylist for tips that will help you keep your hair staying healthy and looking fly.

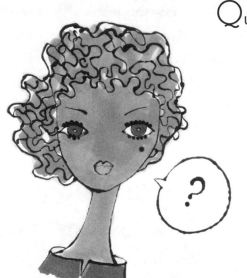

Questions & Answers

Q: I have curly, frizzy hair. Is there some type of product I can use to give it shine? I blow-dry it straight a couple of times a week, and I hate using any product because then my hair doesn't feel clean.

A: The key is finding a product such as a leave-in conditioner that you can use in your hair before you blow-dry it. If there's nothing i n the hair, you're simply burning the natural moisture and oils in your hair. This results in it becoming dry and dull, and it will start to break if it hasn't already.

The rule here for choosing products is that hair that's kinky needs a heavier leave-in conditioner or oil moisturizer. For curly or wavy hair, you should use a light leave-in conditioner. Whichever product is right for you, what you need to keep in mind is to fortify, *fortify* those hair shafts!

Q: I have short, curly hair and I like to wear it straight sometimes. But, when I blow-dry it, it gets this round shape to it. What can I do?

A: Try using a flat (not round) Mason Pearson brush with a mixture of natural and plastic bristles, and start blow-drying your hair when it's wet (not towel dried). Or, simply put a light leave-in conditioner and/or setting lotion on your very wet hair, comb it in the desired direction, and sit under a portable hood dryer until your hair is completely dry.

Q: My hair is thick and kinky and I've been growing it for a couple of years. I'm getting bored with it. Do you have some styling tips for me?

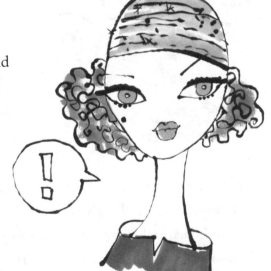

A: Preheat that hood dryer! Try braiding or twisting your hair. With thicker sections you'll get a wavier effect; smaller sections will give you a more crimped effect. Either technique, following a luxurious conditioning treatment, should rev up your creative juices. Have fun!

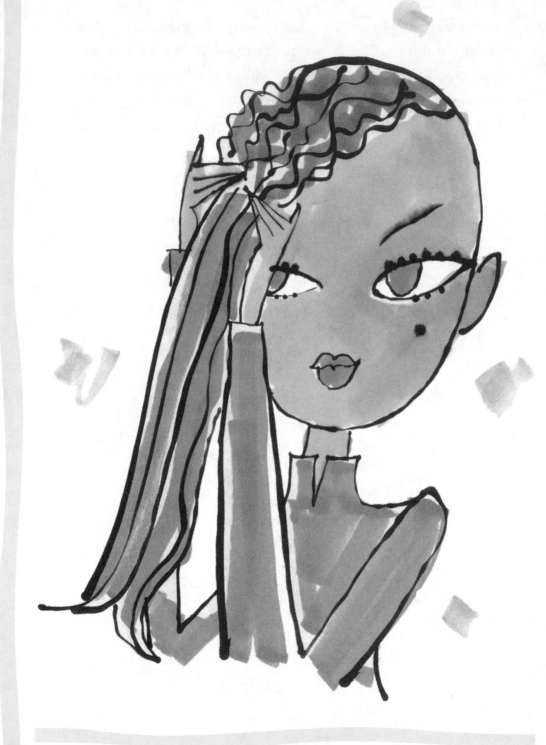

Chapter 5

Relax It!

Should I or Shouldn't I?

I bet you could tell that my byword
is healthy hair! I want you to know
what actually happens to your hair when you
chemically alter its structure and texture.
Knowing what's happening is important,
because you should understand just what
your stylist is doing. That way you can judge
whether her or his methods are good hair care or,
frankly, if you need to move on to someone else. (The more
you know, the better you are at recognizing a good stylist.) I will also explain the various relaxing methods used, and the best ways to take care of
your hair in its chemically altered state.

I have heard many questions about relaxing nonstraight hair during
my eighteen years as a professional hairstylist. My clients have asked me

things like "Can I relax my hair and still maintain some curl?" or, "What kind of relaxers are available for my hair type?" I'm going to try my best to address some of these common concerns.

When it comes to relaxing hair, I think it's important to know some facts about the chemicals that are used. After your hair has been relaxed, it's important to know how to take care of it, so much of the chapter is about what methods of styling and maintenance work best for chemically treated hair.

What it all boils down to is that for many women with kinky or extremely curly hair, the age-old question is whether or not to chemically straighten or texturize (control the curl). Many of my clients have vented their frustrations. They like the styling versatility of straight hair, yet at the same time feel trapped by its high maintenance and the damaging side effects that can occur when their hair is not properly cared for.

C'mon, Ladies, Let's Relax!

Let's first talk about the difference between relaxers and texturizers. Relaxers and texturizers are essentially the same chemical compound. But how they are used and what kinds of hair types they are used on make all the difference in terms of desired results and safety. There are three types of relaxers:

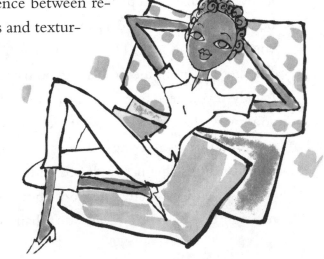

1. *Sodium hydroxide,* commonly called lye, is generally used to relax or texturize the hair. This relaxer can be used for kinky, curly, and wavy hair. Sodium hydroxide requires that your scalp be "based," i.e., coated with a petroleum-based protectant before application that is shampooed out after application.

2. *Calcium hydroxide* is formulated to achieve the same results as sodium hydroxide, but was designed for sensitive scalps. Yet it can be more drying to the hair than sodium hydroxide. Also, this chemical can be more caustic to the scalp if allowed to stay on for too long. Calcium hydroxide, too, can be used for kinky, curly, and wavy hair. The procedure for calcium hydroxide is the same as for sodium hydroxide. First a base is applied to the scalp, and the chemical is washed out afterward.

3. *Ammonium thioglycolate,* the same chemical used for Jheri curls, or curly perms, now comes in a straightening formula. Although it can be used on kinky hair as a presoftener to prepare the hair for a Jheri curl, it's not recommended for straightening or texturizing kinky hair (because it's not a strong enough formula). But it can be used to straighten or texturize curly or wavy hair. Ammonium thioglycolate requires that

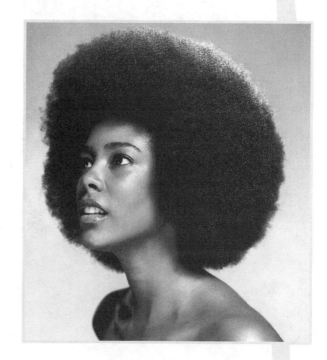

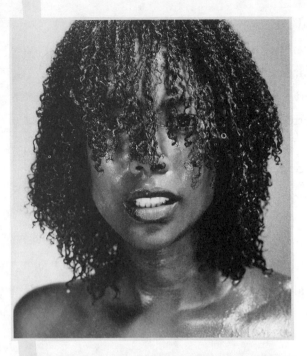

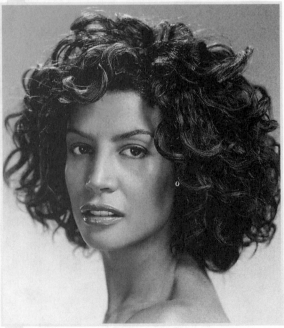

your hair be shampooed *prior* to its application, and not shampooed for at least twenty-four hours after processing. If shampooed before twenty-four hours, your hair will revert to its curly or wavy state.

Thermal Reconditioning

First, don't be fooled by the phrase "reconditioning." This is a chemical straightening process that is fairly new on the market. It is designed for curly to wavy hair types only, and it also contains the chemical ammonium thioglycolate in a low-percentage solution. This process involves using an electric flat iron and is safe for permanently colored hair or hair that has been previously straightened with another ammonium thioglycolate product. Like any new process it has spectacular pros and some dismal cons. In other words, there's good news and there's bad news.

The good news is that thermal reconditioning can transform curly or wavy hair into silky, straight hair with a minimum of damage. The bad news is that, as with any innovative technique, many stylists jump on the bandwagon and proclaim themselves thermal-reconditioning specialists. That seems to justify their charging $500 to $1,000 for an initial treatment. Furthermore, the curlier your hair is, the more often touch-ups are required and, unlike a perm touch-up, you'll wind up paying just as much to recondition any new growth as you did to do your entire head. Here's the arithmetic: Every two to three months you can expect to pay $1,000 to $2,000 for reconditioning treatments alone. If you add to that whatever you typically pay for coloring, cutting, and regular salon visits, that's a hefty price to pay even if you are a diehard straight-styled gal. And did I mention that committing to thermal reconditioning means that you'll have stick-straight hair without an ounce of body?

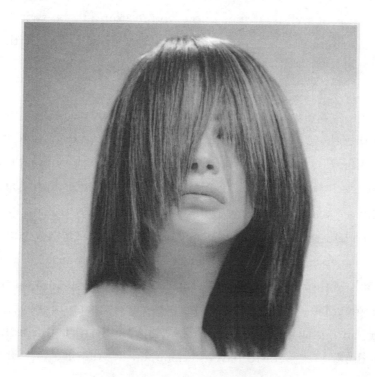

No matter what process you choose, it is in your best interest to be familiar with each of these treatments so that you choose what best suits your hair type and desired style. In choosing any one of these chemical services, it is of the utmost importance to thoroughly understand the commitment involved for your hair and scalp upkeep and maintenance, so by all means, educate yourself and do your research. By the time you consult with your stylist you'll be able to ask some intelligent questions. I realize that this advice may seem weird to many of you who have been straightening your hair for years. Again, I want to remind you that hair science changes and there are improved (and safer) products and techniques to use. What you're used to could very well be obsolete, and your stylist (if she or he keeps up with current trends) may be able to use something better on your hair. Don't you think it's worth finding out?

Speaking of stylists, if you know you're going to be switching hairstylists, make sure you have your former stylist provide you with a record of what method and product was used on your hair. (I know this might be tricky if you're changing stylists because of dissatisfaction, but figure out some way to leave with this information.) The next stylist who does your hair will then have an accurate history of what's been done. He can't necessarily tell just by looking at what's sitting in front of him what kind of relaxer was used on your hair. And while there are some daring artistes out there who are willing to try anything with hair, it's just not advisable when it comes to hair that's been chemically straightened or texturized. The hydroxide relaxers and thioglycolate are not interchangeable. You should never apply either hydroxide to your hair if it's been previously altered with thioglycolate, or vice versa. Mix those and what you'll get is extreme breakage, and what's left of your hair will literally turn to mush. Believe me, you don't ever want to have that happen to you or even see it.

Understanding your hair type and how you want your hair to look is sound preparation for making the commitment to relaxing or texturizing your hair. Remember to be flexible when talking to your stylist with all the information you have. What you see, and what you imagine, may not ultimately be what you should have.

Once you have decided that it is time for a chemical process, you will fall into one of two categories:

1. A woman with natural hair who is seeking more versatility in hair texture, but who fundamentally likes the look and feel of curly or wavy hair and doesn't wish to straighten it, or

2. A woman who already relaxes her hair, and is ready for a touch-up.

If you're in the first category of women, *texturizing* is probably what you'd like, because when done well, it's a subtle enhancement of your hair's natural curl or coil. For those who want to continue with straightened hair, there are some important things to consider about just how to alter your new growth while maintaining your already straightened hair. So, let's take a look.

Texturizing

In texturizing natural hair, a very mild relaxer is used and applied in a careful manner so as not to disturb the hair's natural spring or curl. Depending on the texture you've got and the one you're trying to achieve, it's best if your stylist performs this treatment. Texturizing hair is a delicate procedure. (It's all in the timing.) If you try to do it at home, you run the risk of overstraightening your hair. Slathering and caking the texturizer into hair, or applying it with a large-toothed comb, then leaving it on for too long, have been done by many a do-it-yourselfer. With a pro, when done correctly, texturizing will enhance your hair beautifully by lengthening it and giving your hair a looser curl.

Texturizing can be done with either a mild sodium hydroxide or calcium hydroxide relaxer or an ammonium thioglycolate relaxer. Which to use depends solely on your hair texture. Kinky-spongy or curly-spongy hair, i.e., hair that doesn't have a smooth cuticle, is best texturized using sodium hydroxide or calcium hydroxide. For those of you who have hair that is curly or wavy, ammonium thioglycolate is the most appropriate relaxer to use. Be sure your stylist is aware of the differences for each hair texture because otherwise the results could be devastating.

Your texturized hair should not appear as if it was chemically altered. Instead you should have a natural curl-enhanced effect. Unlike straightened hair, texturized hair needs to be touched up only every three to five months. Infrequent touch-ups are one of many advantages of having texturized hair. Another is the fact that the scalp is less involved, less subject to burning and chemical absorption of potential carcinogens. Many of the problems associated with chemical straightening and damage to one's scalp are minimized when hair is texturized.

Maintenance is a breeze. In fact, texturized hair can be cared for the same as your natural hair. The hair can be rewet, reconditioned, and, with a little styling lotion, conditioning gel, foam, or a nice fragrant essential oil, styled as often as desired. Your texturized hair should be air-dried or dried under a portable hood dryer. What could be simpler than that?

•   •   •

Chemical Straightening

If you're chemically straightening your hair, take heed of the upkeep and commitment involved with such an extreme permanent process. You're taking your hair to its absolute max and because of that, you need to be disciplined with your maintenance routine. Skin and other body tissues absorb chemicals, allowing them to get into your bloodstream and increasing the risk of exposure to carcinogens. It's highly recommended that shampooing not be done for one full week prior to getting your hair chemically straightened. This is recommended so that the scalp can accumulate as much oil as possible to protect itself from the toxic effect of sodium hydroxide or the thioglycolate. (This is an additional precaution used along with basing the scalp with a petroleum protectant.) The body and scalp are susceptible to dermatitis, so make sure your scalp is liberally based before applying any chemical relaxers.

Handle with Loving Care

Touch-ups, the relaxing of new growth, must be done with meticulous care. I do not recommend that touch-ups be done at home. Professionals are best for this delicate procedure. Touch-ups can cause severe damage and breakage to previously relaxed hair, particularly around the hairline and the nape of the neck. Take note and be concerned about any stylist who is cheerfully applying chemical relaxer beyond your new growth. (As a matter of fact, the first time you go to a stylist, go early. See how she or he works with hair similar to yours. If she gets slap-happy with the relaxer and spends more time chatting up the client than paying attention to how much and where she is placing relaxer, I suggest you start talking into your cell phone as if your kids just called to tell you they've set the house on fire, and then get the hell out of that salon!)

Hair relaxed straight should be shampooed once a week, deep conditioned, and wet set. If you're an active woman who works out, be sure to wear a terry-cloth sweatband along your hairline while you're at the gym or health club. Afterward, a light blow-dry on cool with your comb attachment is permissible. For the regular styling of relaxed hair, I recommend wet setting, or wrapping the hair with a light setting lotion and blow-drying it on low to medium heat only. If you have a short Halle Berry cut, it can be a breeze. Just wrap and go.

Remember earlier I said that relaxing is an extreme process? What that means in real terms is that your hair is now more fragile and drier than it was. That's true whether you have thick hair or thin hair, coarse or fine. The point is, if you have hair, it's now in a more vulnerable state. Handle with care. Before you use a hot comb or a curling iron to style your hair, consider that you're literally playing with fire! Ultimately what you'll end up with is extremely damaged, broken hair. Think about it: If you're going to use all that heat on your hair, why would you relax it straight in the first place? Keep the high heat for unstraightened hair. (It can take the stress better.) Instead, learn how to wet set your hair to achieve a beautiful style.

That's one of the reasons I've written an entire chapter on the virtues of wet setting. Thanks to wet setting you can have beautifully relaxed hair and style it however you like, all the while minimizing the risk of long-term damage. If that's not win-win, I don't know what is!

I recommend that you treat your scalp after every touch-up or chemical service with essential oils such as comfrey, peppermint, tea tree, or

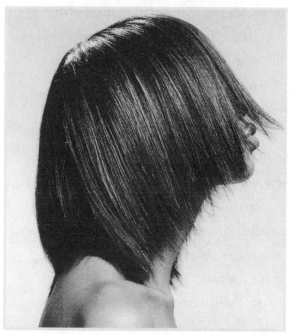

horsetail. Their soothing, astringent properties are a great boost to your hair and scalp's general well-being. Using light essential oils after a chemical process serves to remind you that they have been subjected to a demanding treatment, and helps to balance out some of the stress. You can find most of these oils in health food stores.

For all chemically straightened or texturized hair, I can't stress enough that it's best to sleep with a satin scarf or pillowcase. Cotton absorbs oil and frizzes the hair. Allowing your hair to get frizzy defeats the purpose of all the massaging and conditioning you're committed to doing, right?

All that I've shared with you in this chapter is to help you be a more mindful consumer and caretaker of your hair. With this information, and armed with some great tips in terms of your choices, your chemical experience can be a spectacular success.

•   •   •

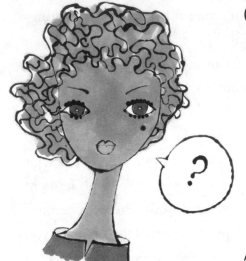

Questions & Answers

Q: I have hair that's chemically straightened and I see a dermatologist for a bald spot. My hairstylist and my dermatologist tell me that my bald spot is not getting any better. What should I do?

A: I won't beat around the bush. Find a new way to get a straight-haired look (such as a weave or a wig) or go natural. You implied that you, your doctor, and your stylist are all alarmed about your bald spot. Yet which of the two of them is going to blow the whistle and tell you what you probably don't want to hear: *Stop!*?

Whatever you're doing to your hair when it's being straightened is happening to your scalp, too. Memorize this formula: chemicals + skin = burns. Give your hair and scalp a rest.

Q: I think I'm able to handle relaxing my hair at home, especially now that there are the no-lye products on the market. Any advice?

A: First off, even the no-lye relaxers (which usually contain calcium hydroxide) can do damage to your hair and scalp. I particularly want you to be mindful of the stress on your scalp because of the repeated applications of a caustic solution. The strength or percentage of the active product in chemical relaxers should be adjusted for each person's hair texture and desired results. That's not something you're going to be able to do at home.

Also, depending on where you are in your life cycle, your hair's texture can change. Factors such as pregnancy, or high stress, or even age affect what kind of hair you have and its overall condition. An off-the-shelf relaxer kit is "one size fits all." Look, even over-the-counter medicines have suggested dosages based on age. Wouldn't you think that relaxers would need similar limits based, at the very least, on a woman's hair type and texture?

Another reason I don't think it's a good idea to relax your hair at home is because of a common misconception that you may share with many hairstylists that the kinkier the hair, the coarser it is. Such an error in judgment can cause a stylist to use too strong a chemical on the hair, which often results in overprocessed hair. If a professional can make a mistake like that, can't you?

It's the possibility of abusing your hair and scalp that concerns me. That's why Dr. Downie and I are adamant in insisting that relaxing should be done by a competent professional, and at the first sign of any problems, you should seek professional help. Once the hair or the scalp have been damaged, they cannot be returned to a normal, healthy state without intervention.

Look, the last thing I want for you in your pursuit of beauty is that you become a Rogaine candidate later on in life. Sometimes there is nothing (short of a very, very expensive hair transplant and/or weave) that can be done that will give you a full head of hair. And, for many of you, that's not a realistic option.

Q: I want to get my hair texturized now. Currently, I wear it relaxed. How can I make the transition from that to a texturized style?

A: The short answer is: You can't. Chemically straightened hair is permanent, and you won't be able to alter the hair's essential straightness other than by styling techniques. While I sympathize with your wish to have a curlier hairstyle, you simply mustn't add texturizer to straightened hair. (Remember, by relaxing your hair you've already taken your hair to its max.)

However, there are a few different ways you can approach going back to a look that more resembles your natural hair. You can get a spiral set (hair rolled on rods or straws) while your hair is growing out, or you can wear a weave or braids while growing out the relaxer. If you're really game, let your hair grow one to two inches, cut off the relaxed hair, and then have the virgin growth texturized.

If you decide to try braids, which is very common as one of today's fashionable hair statements, be sure that your braid technician doesn't pull your braids too tight. Let her or him know the moment it feels tight. Over time constant pulling can cause *folliculitis, traction alopecia,* hair thinning, and/or breakage. (In Chapter 8, Dr. Downie talks about the damage that can be done to a woman's hair and scalp by wearing tight hairstyles.)

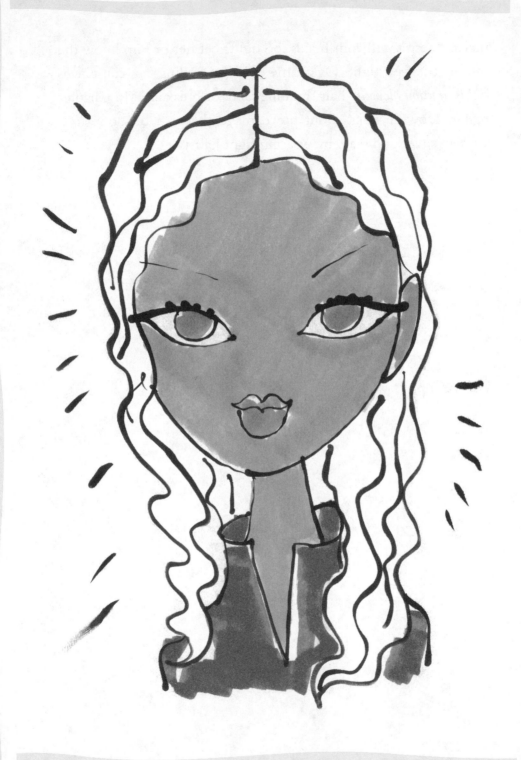

Chapter 6

Color It!

What Did You Do to Look So New?

When a woman decides to color
her hair, especially a permanent change, there are some
important things to con-
sider. This chapter out-
lines the pros and cons of
coloring with permanent
and semipermanent colors
and rinses. I want to awaken
you to the possibilities available
to you in the world of hair color. You
can change your look by lightening or darkening
your hair in less than one hour. The important thing is to have fun with
your color change. It will look great as long as you follow certain rules

when you do this to your hair. This is especially true if your hair is already chemically relaxed or texturized.

Hair coloring has gone through many changes. Not so long ago, doing it was the big secret women kept to themselves. Remember "Does she or doesn't she?" Fortunately, times have changed, and hair coloring has come out of the closet, with home hair coloring becoming more popular than ever. Now almost 50 percent of women of all ages color their hair, either to disguise gray or as a fashion accessory. And why not? Coloring has the power to transform and enhance a woman's beauty by complementing her skin color and complexion, and adding depth and luster to her hair.

Louis Licari and I strongly recommend starting out consulting with a professional colorist who can answer some of your questions and lead you in the right direction. In fact, if you're thinking of getting your hair colored for the very first time, *please* have it done by a professional colorist. Seeing a professional makes hair coloring easy. He or she will look at your hair and make suggestions on what would be best for you, taking into consideration your hair type, texture, and condition. Most hair colorists are masters of illusion, and have developed an application of color that can't be mimicked or matched by off-the-shelf colors.

I understand that going to a salon is a great luxury. If you can't afford to spend the time or money to go to the salon regularly, try to go at least once or twice a year to keep your color on the right track. (There are many things the back of the color box won't teach you.) Also, once you've colored your hair, a good hair-care regimen needs to be followed religiously. Your colorist can answer your questions about how to care for your newly colored hair.

Dramatic color changes require the help of a professional but more

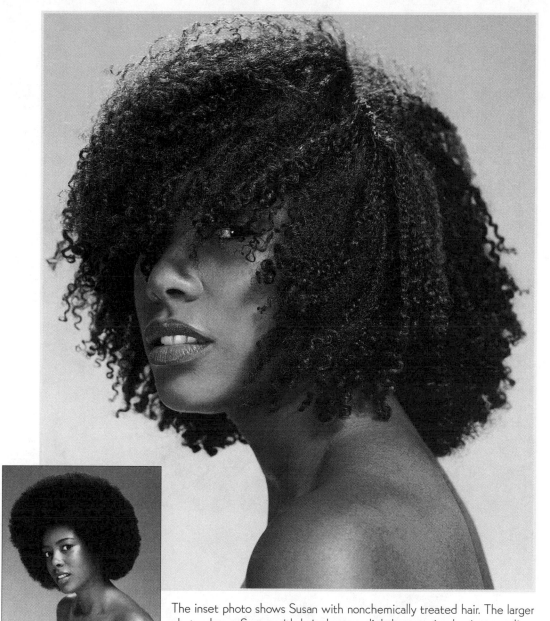

The inset photo shows Susan with nonchemically treated hair. The larger photo shows Susan with hair that was lightly texturized using a sodium hydroxide relaxer. We were then able to take her hair color a stage further by both lightening her base and adding highlights. If we had chosen to relax Susan's hair completely straight we couldn't have done multiple stages of color without doing damage to her hair.

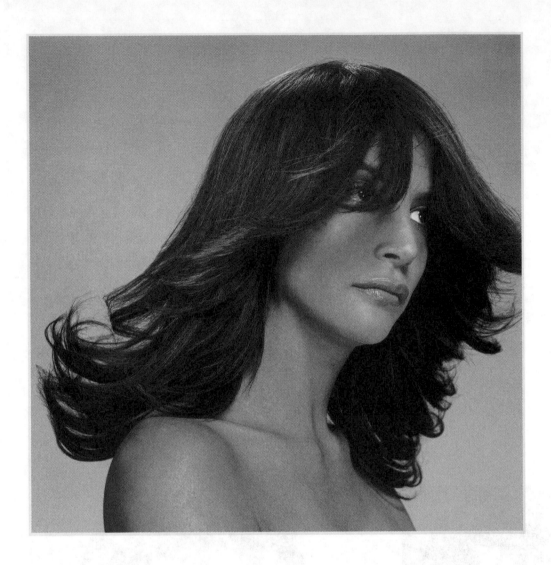

Kara actually has shoulder-length hair, but we added sixteen inches with a sewn-in weave. We then razored the hair, which allows it all to blend naturally.

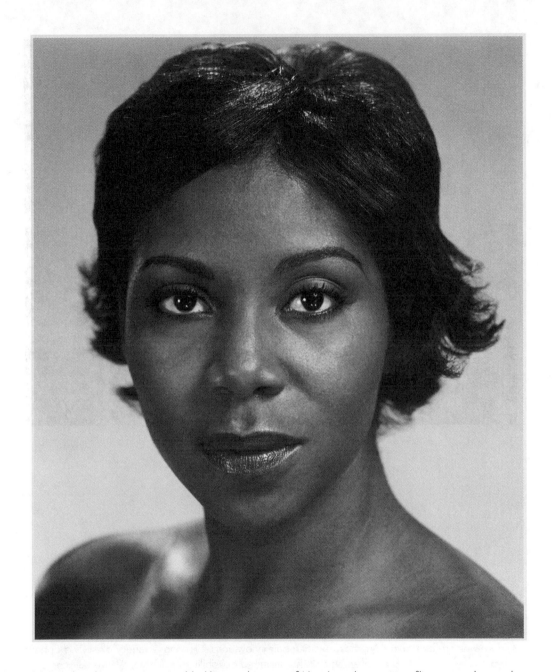

Using a bonding process, we added hair to the nape of Nona's neck, creating a flip to complement her short pixie cut.

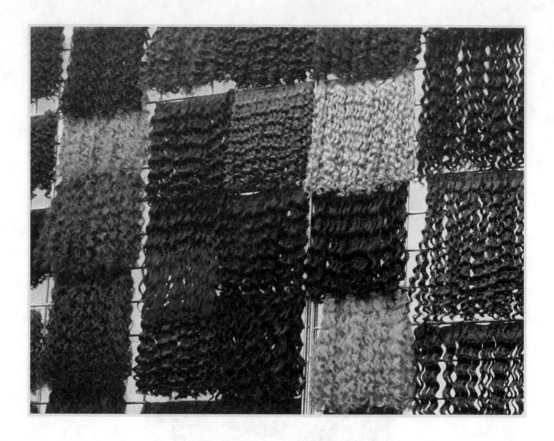

Hair weaves are one of today's most exciting hair innovations, offering a variety of styling options to women who dare to take advantage of the unlimited possibilities available. Weave hair comes in various colors and grades (kinky, curly, wavy, silky, etc.), and good-quality hair is an investment. Have fun with it!

subtle color changes can be achieved with at-home color. At-home color works. The tip here is to stay within two shades of your natural color. This will prevent strong regrowth lines. Going lighter will soften and warm your hair color. Going darker will add depth and make your color rich. Remember, hair color should always provide contrast with skin color. It will make your skin color come alive. When your new color is right, you will find you won't have to wear as much makeup.

The results of today's colors are predictable, especially when you do a strand test. This is when you apply the chosen color to a section of your hair from the nape area. The color that section becomes is the color you are going to achieve.

Highlighting

Highlighting is another option for curly or kinky hair. This is a favorite because the highlights will help to define the curls. It's entirely up to you whether you want to choose a color that looks natural or one that is a bit extreme. Whatever your decision, you should have a touch-up every three to four months. Here are some highlighting tips:

1. If what you're striving for is a natural look, make sure the highlight color relates to your natural color base. For instance, if you have dark golden-brown hair, you want to choose a dark golden highlight.

2. Go slow. You can always add more highlights later. You don't have to use the whole package at once!

3. Always use tint highlights rather than bleach highlights. They are more gentle and compatible with chemically serviced hair.

4. Highlights don't have to start at the scalp. This means you can chemically texturize or straighten regrowth without overlapping relaxer on colored hair.

All in all, color helps to create a look as much as styling does. You can start with color and make your look unique to you. Have fun with it! You will love the new you.

From Temporary to Permanent

You'll be doing yourself a big favor, if you're thinking about coloring your hair, by consulting a professional colorist. When it comes to the exciting possibilities offered by coloring your hair, Louis and I both realize the powerful lure of do-it-yourself hair coloring. Many women like to use over-the-counter hair rinses and dyes to jazz up their own color. The effects of the colors in the stores, despite the labels of *temporary, semipermanent,* and *permanent,* cannot be predicted as accurately as the labels would lead you to believe. The strength of

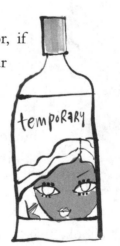
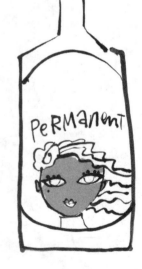

a coloring product depends on the amount of peroxide in the solution. Peroxide works as a pigment activator, opening up the hair cuticle and making it possible for the color to be deposited and the hair shaft to absorb the pigment. The amount of peroxide can vary from manufacturer to manufacturer. Despite those variations, there are three basic types of hair color:

Temporary hair colors are simple rinses that contain certified food colors that coat the hair's cuticle. They don't penetrate the shaft, and are great after a chemical straightening to add shine and luster to the hair. Temporary rinses are just that, temporary. The color will fade each time you shampoo. However, for women with kinky hair, the truth of the matter is that if your hair is gray or white, there's no such thing as temporary hair color. I've got news for you, girlfriend: Temporary hair color will permanently stain your hair. Once you apply any pigment to it, you've permanently colored the hair. In fact, the whiter and lighter your grays are, the more it will stain. This is something to think about if you have graying hair and are flirting with the idea of going all the way with hair color.

Semipermanent hair color also coats the hair, but some contain a small percentage of peroxide and can deposit color or an activator. Activators add the boost that gives the color its staying power. The activator penetrates the cuticle. A lot of off-the-shelf box color comes with an activator that makes the resulting hair color darker. Understand that while advertisements claim it's temporary, even so, you might end up with a deeper shade than you expected or desired. If you keep in mind that any semipermanent color you apply will be darker than your natural hair color, your expectations of the kind of look you can achieve will be more realistic.

A lot of women prefer semipermanent color because it does cover gray with more staying power. The color can last four to eight weeks.

Unless gray hairs are starting to show through any previously colored ends, you don't need to apply the color from root to end. Instead, concentrate on coloring the roots. Otherwise, you might get a buildup of color on the ends, which will make them appear noticeably darker than the rest of your hair.

Color buildup is a telltale sign of a poorly done coloring job. In nature, most of you (unless your new hair grows out gray) have darker roots than ends. You want to approximate nature's paintbrush when you use semipermanent color.

Permanent hair color is combined with 20 percent or more of peroxide. This type of color is for women who have more than 20 percent gray hair or want a more dramatic change in their appearance. Permanent hair coloring should be done only to healthy hair that is in its natural state, or hair that has been only lightly chemically texturized. If your hair has been chemically straightened, the percentage of peroxide should be lowered to between 10 and 15 percent. In fact, here's a tip for all you ladies out there with chemically altered hair: adding one-quarter to one-half ounce of water to your hair-coloring solution will reduce its peroxide strength. Not lowering the percentage of peroxide could result in severe damage. This is exactly why home perm kits warn consumers not to use the product if their hair has been bleached. Remember this: You can color your hair and you can relax your hair, but take caution when doing both together.

Any chemical relaxing should be done at least one week before coloring. This will help you choose the right color for the condition of your hair. It is best to keep the coloring as gentle as possible when dealing with relaxed hair. Be sure to leave permanent hair color to the professionals, because the long-term beauty of permanent hair coloring depends so much on the hair's prior condition, its upkeep, and maintenance. It takes a lot of work to keep permanently colored hair that's been relaxed looking its best. Many women insist on altering the texture of their hair after it's been colored. If that's what you prefer, so be it, but let a good stylist take the lead in keeping your hair healthy.

Shampooing and Conditioning

Whatever the reasons for a woman with nonstraight hair to add color, it's always important that the hair be in good condition. Now that you know what happens when you color your hair, particularly the interaction of color with chemically treated hair, you're more apt to approach the entire process with good sense. When shampooing and conditioning colored hair, treat your hair as though it were *extremely* dry and use the appropriate products and procedures that I talked about in Chapters 2 and 3. For chemically treated hair that's been colored, focus on cleaning your scalp only, and condition your hair with a vengeance once a week.

After all, color is your hottest hair accessory, and despite my warnings, I say go for it.

• • •

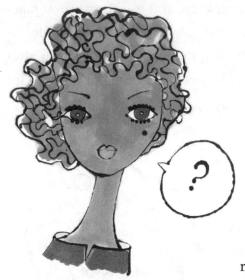

Questions & Answers

Q: I have highlights, which I love. What do I do now that my roots are growing out?

A: For that in-between stage, I suggest that you add highlights to lighten just your roots instead of reapplying highlights to the rest of your hair. Doing just the new growth is gentler on the hair.

Q: I chemically relax my hair and I want to color it myself. What's the best color to use?

A: I encourage you to seek out a professional, particularly because your hair is relaxed straight. Certainly for the first time, at least. The colorist may be able to use a gentler product on your hair and advise you on what over-the-counter products you can use thereafter to maintain both your color and your hair's health.

Q: I straighten my hair and it's getting lighter and kind of dull. What type of color do you suggest I use?

A: A temporary rinse will work just fine. It will make your own hair stronger and shinier because it acts like a filler for your hair's cuticles and smooths them down. And it does all that—color, strengthen, and add shine—without any additional chemicals.

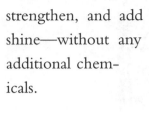

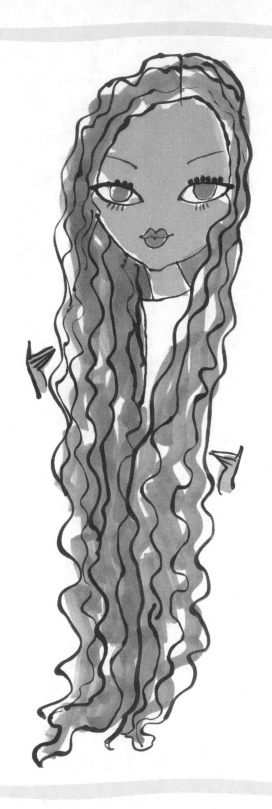

Chapter 7

"Unbeweavable"

To Weave or Not to Weave?

Hair extensions (hair braided or bonded onto half-centimeter sections of one's own hair), weaves (a weft of hair sewn onto a corn-row), and bonding (a weft of hair glued to the scalp) are today's most exciting hair innovations.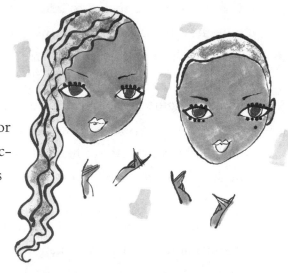

Techniques that were once the province of trendsetters and the professionally chic, e.g., models and actresses, are now for you. What is revolutionary about these new hair additions is that they offer a variety of styling options for women who dare to take advantage of the unlimited possibilities available. For instance, a natural style can be easily transformed into a long, straight 'do, or even a short, Halle Berry–like style, without chemically straightening the hair. Or, say you're growing out a relaxer and are undecided as to how to wear your hair, but you're certainly not interested in having short hair: A curly, wavy weave at any length may suffice. Better yet, you can also change your color without affecting your natural color.

Some women add hair for a fuller look, some add length, and others may want a bang or perhaps a flip. Some women want to add hair to cover up badly damaged hair. Whatever the reason, there's no excuse for walking down the street with a rug on your head (unless, of course, you're moving and that's how you carry your prized possessions). So many beautiful women do just that. Why? They may not know any better.

Remember the old saying "It takes money to make money?" Well, the same principle applies to getting a weave. What I mean by that is that it takes healthy hair to add healthy hair. So, if you want to get a weave because your hair's a mess, I have one word for you: *Don't!* A bad weave is one that has been attached to badly damaged hair, like a beautiful lipstick trying to disguise a mouthful of rotten teeth.

If your hair is already weak or overprocessed from relaxers and/or coloring, or your scalp is inflamed, then a weave is not advisable. If this is you, stop here and read Dr. Downie's advice in Chapter 8. A weave might get in the way of restoring your own hair to health. There may be a better intermediate-style solution available to you. In the meantime, with diligence and patience, your hair will become healthier, and this chapter will be waiting for you. I promise.

You'd Better Shop Around

Good-quality hair is an investment. Purchasing the proper human hair is as important a step as any to having a natural-looking weave. Hair comes in a number of grades: kinky, curly, silky, and wavy, to name a few. Those grades come already prepared, colored, and sewn into a weft (hair segments sewn to a woven band) and ready to be applied. You can also go in and have the hair professionally matched to your own grade and texture of hair. There are places called "hair factories" where you select the texture and color of your choice. The hair is assembled on-site and sewn into a customized weft for you.

No matter what grade is used, the hair is refined by chemicals and processed for the retailer, i.e., it is made more pliable for coloring and achieving desired textures. How healthy and strong the donor hair is determines how well it will withstand any chemical and/or coloring processes, as well as any manufacturing processes. Good-quality hair may cost a little more, but you will make out better in the long run because you won't be purchasing hair every six to eight weeks. It can be reused for six months or so—not worn continuously, mind you, but reapplied. It also looks more natural as it is reused if it is properly cared for and maintained. Good-quality hair is like the difference between Gucci and the Gap. You do get what you pay for.

Your stylist should always have a good source for purchasing excellent-quality hair. If she or he doesn't, consider waiting until she or he does, or go elsewhere. It makes a big difference. Use common sense when purchasing hair; if you have fine hair, you don't want to purchase a thick or coarse grade of hair. Always be sure to select the texture of hair closest to your own. Also, be sure the new hair is washed and conditioned to remove the chemical residue and smell.

I'm assuming your stylist is someone in whom you have complete confidence. You should be comfortable talking candidly with him or her about your desired style. (If not, take a look at Chapter 1 for my tips on how to find the right stylist.) Be especially careful that your stylist doesn't braid your hair too tightly, as it will cause permanent hair loss. You want a good job done technically, but if it's not your style, what good will it do you or your pocketbook? So again, don't be shy about making your styling needs clear.

Care and Maintenance

Once the hair is attached, weekly salon visits or home care is essential to maintain your investment. Care begins with shampooing the scalp thoroughly. Do this gently to avoid loosen-

ing, tangling, or matting the weave. Squeezing is best. Be sure to use an ultramoisturizing shampoo and always use a liberal amount of conditioner.

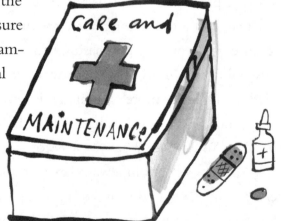

Every six to eight weeks the weave should be removed. You heard me: Get it out! After you've gone through all this trouble to make your hair look so realistic, you may forget that your own hair and scalp need to breathe. Relieve the stress on your hair and scalp by giving them at least one full week of rest. I suggest you sport a smart ponytail for a while. Remember, one of your primary reasons for having a weave is that you desire longer, fuller hair. Therefore, hair and scalp treatments are a must, otherwise—how can I put it?—you won't have any hair to attach there.

Bonding

Did someone say bonding? Instant enhancement. Bonding is a temporary technique to achieve a quick, "gotta go" style. Glue is first applied to the weft of hair. (Let me caution you that bonding glue consists of rubber-based materials, and some of you may experience an immediate allergic reaction to the glue. If that's the case, stop immediately and remove the glue following the steps I describe below.) Then the weft is applied to a clean scalp. This bonding glue breaks down when it comes in contact with oil, so, depending on your own scalp's oil level, a bonded weave will usually last three to five days, at most a week.

When it's time to remove the weave, I recommend using a scalp oil or silicone spray. It is the most effective method for removing glue from your scalp and hair. It should be sprayed directly on the weft and scalp. Saturate both thoroughly. Massage the scalp gently and let the oil or silicone stay in long enough to soften the glue. (Don't tear at the weft; wait until the glue softens. After that, the weft should slide out effortlessly.) With a fine-toothed comb remove the remaining glue from your scalp and hair. Add more oil or silicone spray to your hair, if needed. Don't be stingy with the oil or silicone. Leftover glue can lead to hair and scalp damage, so make sure you get it all out. Since bonding itself is temporary (let's say it's a preliminary to getting a weave, an easy way to try out a look), don't waste your money on expensive hair.

Let me be clear here: I do not rule out outrageous color and style. I trust you know your own personal style, and that's where yaky hair comes into play. What is yaky hair? It's inexpensive, refined, and processed human hair combined with yak fur—yes, yak fur—cleverly disguised to become the texture and color of your choice. Yaky hair comes in textures that range from deep wave to straw, and shades from pumpkin orange to bright magenta to carrot-top red. The hair has an almost synthetic feel to it. I suggest using it for a party look, or a temporary hairstyle. Discard yaky hair after one or two cycles of usage.

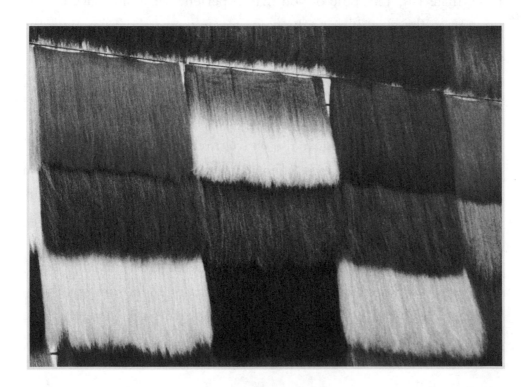

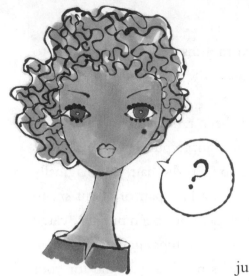

Questions & Answers

Q: My hair is fine and lay-
ered to chin length. I'd like
to have hair down to my
shoulders. What should I
do?

A: I'm assuming your hair is
just fine naturally, and not fine from
split ends, breakage, overcoloring, and/or
chemical relaxing. If so, your hair would be a perfect candidate for
two or three wefts of hair: at the temples and nape of the neck.
Make sure to keep in line with your existing cut, and make sure to
have your new weave razor cut to your desired length.

Q: I have a soft, kinky natural cut that I've worn out in an Afro, in
cornrows, twists—you name it. I'm tempted to cut it and relax it
straight. But relaxing it is what led me to growing it out natural,
and I'm so enjoying the low maintenance of my natural. What
now?

A: *What!* Now calm down and get a weave. Pick a color, any color,
and a texture other than European silky straight. Perhaps relaxed
straight hair would better suit you, keeping in mind that African-
American women have much more texture to their hair, and realistic is what you are going for with the weave. Now feel free to
cut, color, curl, and what have you!

Q: I had my weave put in about two months ago and I'm going to have it redone. Should I expect to pay the same amount?

A: First of all, your weave should have been removed two weeks ago. Six weeks is the maximum time you want to put that kind of stress on your scalp and hair. Second, as long as the hair you originally purchased was of good quality, it has a life span of about six to eight months from the time of purchase. If it's been properly cared for, it can be reapplied. Since you're not purchasing new hair, you shouldn't expect to pay your stylist as much as you did for your first application. (Unless, of course, you purchased the hair yourself the first time.) I'll let you do the math: With prudent care, this weave can be reapplied a few more times before it's necessary to purchase a new one.

Q: I have a short, pixie cut and enjoy having short hair, but there's this new style I saw in a magazine similar to mine except it had a little flip in the back and small bangs. Am I asking too much?

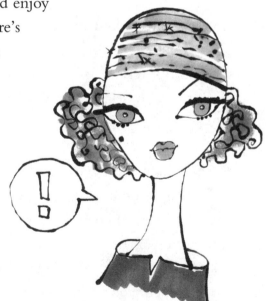

A: I swear, most new hair innovations were brought about by clients and their sometimes over-the-top requests. Of course that's not too much to ask! Did someone say bonding? With a little bonding glue on a track of hair your color match, snip here and razor there, and you've got a quick, temporary style to go in no time. Just make sure your stylist is up to it.

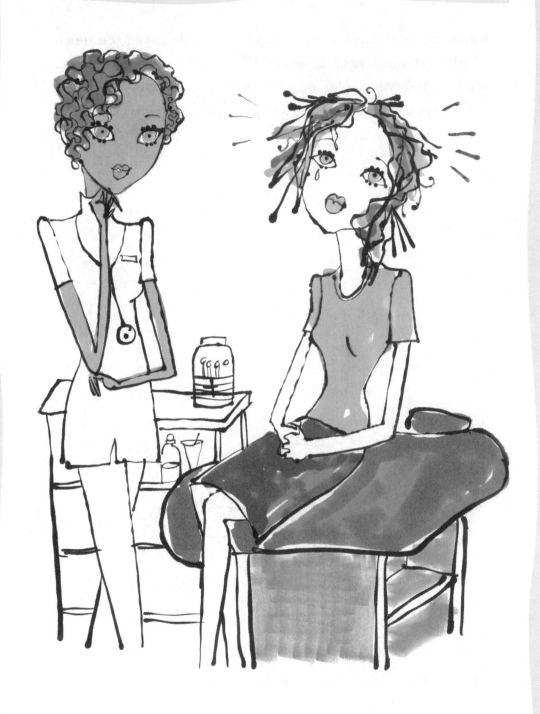

Chapter 8

The Doctor Can See You Now

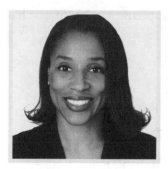

Meet Dr. Jeanine Downie

Jeanine B. Downie, MD, is a dermatologist with extensive experience in hair loss and diseases and disorders of the scalp. Because the state of your hair and scalp can reflect a serious medical issue, she is always on the lookout for any underlying conditions. Yet in her practice Dr. Downie spends considerable time advising her patients about appropriate hair care in general, in addition to hair care when in treatment for a medical condition.

After several years seeing women who suffer from preventable or manageable hair and scalp problems, Dr. Downie is a fervent advocate of a four-square strategy of patient education, good nutrition, overall fitness, and professional hair care. This approach, in her estimation, is the best long-term insurance for any woman who wants to maintain a healthy head of hair.

Many of her patients and my clients share common concerns for their hair. Often we are asked questions about hair loss, thinning, lack of growth, and problems originating from relaxing or coloring the hair. The doctor and I talked at length about these all-too-familiar occurrences. Here she provides some candid and often surprising answers to when and why to see a dermatologist for your hair, general hair care, and the enduring myths about nonstraight hair. She goes on to discuss the roles pregnancy, physical and mental well-being, genetics, and disease play in your hair's (and scalp's) appearance. Here is what she has to say:

Dermatology

D: What's the difference between a trichologist and a dermatologist?

JD: A person who calls her- or himself a trichologist is usually a beautician, cosmetologist, or stylist who has studied hair science at a holistic center. All hairstylists are not trichologists, but most trichologists have been professional hairstylists. Many stylists become trichologists due to their years of experience working with normal and abnormal hair conditions. Trichologists are often affiliated with hair salons, and a woman may be referred to a trichologist by a salon or a dermatologist. A dermatologist is a medical doctor, someone who has successfully completed four years of medical school and a four-year dermatology residency studying medical and cosmetic issues regarding hair, skin, nails, and the mucous membranes (lips and genitalia).

In my practice, depending on what a patient is being treated for, I often refer her to a trichologist and a professional hairstylist. Just because a woman has a serious or severe scalp condition doesn't mean that she should stop being concerned about her appearance. (In fact, most of my patients can't afford to!) Therefore, a referral to a professional stylist, someone who can work with my patient's hair, and is knowledgeable and mindful of the medical condition and treatment used, is a valuable partner in a treatment plan. It makes sense: If a patient is faced with a months-long or even year-long course of treatment, attractive grooming by an expert is strong motivation. A person who is inspired by her ability to still keep up appearances is a person who is more willing to abide by the treatment regimen with patience and discipline.

D: Why should a woman go to a dermatologist when she is having trouble with her scalp and/or hair?

JD: If a woman is experiencing hair loss it may be from a number of things. Hair loss can be caused by a specific disease or disorder, but, in many instances, hair loss, whether breakage or thinning, is usually caused by excessive or improper grooming, as is the case with overdyeing, self-perming, glue from adding extensions, and a lack of trimming and conditioning.

Family history, too, is an important factor: *androgenetic alope-cia,* i.e., male-pattern baldness, is also high on the list of reasons women are experiencing hair loss. Where there is no underlying medical condition, a woman can be referred to a trichologist or a stylist.

However, hair loss and scalp conditions can be symptomatic of other problems. A woman should go to a dermatologist when she is having trouble with her scalp and/or hair in order to rule out *fungus* and any underlying medical conditions, such as diabetes, thyroid problems, anemia, and, less commonly, *lupus* and *lichenplanopilaris.* It is very important to see a dermatologist if a woman suffers from specific skin conditions such as *seborrheic dermatitis* (dandruff) or *psoriasis,* which may not always be localized on the scalp.

Finally, if the suspected reason for hair loss is related to stress (as in the case of *alopecia areata,* discussed in detail later), it's important that a woman see both a dermatologist and a hairstylist. Working in tandem, both professionals can help treat stress-related hair loss.

D: What should a person know when choosing a dermatologist?

JD: When choosing a dermatologist, a woman should get a referral from someone who has been or is a satisfied patient. Keep in mind that since there is a mind-body connection between your mental health and the appearance of your skin, you may wind up being treated by a dermatologist for something that involves disclosing sensitive aspects of your life. You'll need to be comfortable enough with your dermatologist to be able to be forthright about any stressors that may have an impact.

For a dermatologist, the condition of a woman's hair and scalp can provide some preliminary clues to her problem. But no biopsy or microscopic examination of hair will reveal to the doctor that a person's going through the agonies of divorce or is losing a job. Be prepared to share with your dermatologist any emotional problems, for the success of the regimen ultimately decided upon is related to the problem's root causes.

Don't go to a dermatologist expecting magic. It takes intimate cooperation between you and your doctor if one of the causes of hair loss is linked to emotional factors. Be sure the dermatologist you choose is someone you feel you can form a bond with, in addition to making sure that the person whose expertise you're seeking is board-certified.

Also, for an initial standard consultation, start with no more than two main issues that you want to focus on and address.

D: When should a person consider seeking professional medical help?

JD: Most people wouldn't dream of seeing a dermatologist for a mild case of dandruff, and I wouldn't blame them. However, there are some rules of thumb as to when it might be advisable to seek professional help. If that mild case of dandruff (or any other troubling condition) persists and gets worse despite conscientious use of over-the-counter treatments, it's time to see a dermatologist. If there is a particular condition, or certain diseases where there's a strong family history, again it's advisable to see a dermatologist. I repeat, some scalp conditions are indicative of serious illnesses, and should be checked out, not ignored.

D: Are you encountering diseases or conditions in your practice now that you didn't encounter years ago?

JD: In the past five years that I've been in private practice, I'm seeing more females with hair in places they do not want it, such as on chins and faces, as well as more female baldness. Some of this can be attributed to the presence of hormones, specifically androgens, in nonorganic chicken, other meats, and dairy products. This is why many dermatologists are encouraging their patients to eat organically. More young women are coming to me with hairy chins (something that we typically didn't see until middle age and the elder years) and, as I mentioned previously, more mature women are experiencing male-pattern baldness.

D: Are treatments and medications for scalp and hair disorders covered by most insurance plans?

JD: In general, yes, although the insurance companies are trying to classify many treatments and medications as cosmetic. If there is any question, the best bet is for a woman to check with her individual plan.

Best Practices: What You as a Dermatologist Would Advise Any Woman

D: Are there any over-the-counter hair products or therapies that you consider harmful? Are there any products and processes that you'd advise your patients to avoid?

JD: I'm a strong opponent of self-perming and self-coloring. However, it's unrealistic for me to expect people to stop self-perming and -coloring, just because I consider these practices potentially harmful. If a woman insists on doing it herself, I urge her to follow the package instructions faithfully. Often what women do is perm or color the hair when it is in poor condition. Or, dissatisfied with the results of a perm or a coloring job, follow up closely with another perm or another dye job. All I can say is: I'll be seeing you (or a professional stylist will)! The probability of your hair breaking or your scalp burning is very high.

Another area that I want to caution hair-product users about is overseas products. Few nations have an FDA that has rigorous standards for what we humans can apply or ingest. Therefore, some hair-care products coming out of Africa, the Caribbean, Europe, and South America contain unsafe portions of mercury or steroids. Don't take any chances. This is one time when buying American is not just patriotic, but a smart personal health decision. It goes without saying that any product that has the potential to harm an adult has increased potential to do harm to a developing fetus.

D: Are there any over-the-counter hair products or therapies that you consider ineffective?

JD: I think that a woman is getting what she pays for when she uses two-in-one conditioning shampoos. You're getting a half-price shampoo and you're getting a half-price conditioner, and the value to your hair will be just about halved, too. Shampoo and conditioner have different purposes, and are formulated to work in tandem, not simultaneously. The same holds true for combination conditioner/styling products. What you gain in convenience you lose in efficacy.

The emphasis on natural products can sometimes lead people to purchase products whose utility has no basis in fact. Just because something is *natural* doesn't mean that it is effective. So, some prudence should be used. Many people swear by *biotin,* which is said to improve hair thickness. My position on biotin is this: As of yet it seems to do no harm. If any of my patients use it, or want to, I won't discourage it. But I will say that in terms of ingesting vitamins, a person is better off taking a daily multivitamin. Hair is affected by one's overall nourishment. The hair itself doesn't need special vitamins.

I'm sure you've wistfully heard of or read all about the

hair-loss pills, solutions, and regimens that are advertised on the radio and at the back of magazines. Their claims are typically never based in reality. Hair loss is a serious condition that can be the result of many interconnected factors: general health, genetics, poor hair-care habits, etc. There are no magic pills or solutions that can counteract any factor that has caused someone to lose her hair. If there were, I'd be prescribing them and working one tenth as hard as I do now for my patients. Let me amend that a bit, because there is Rogaine, and while it isn't magical, it can be very effective for some patients. I'd be happy to talk more about using Rogaine as a viable hair-replacement option.

D: If a woman can't afford to see a physician, are there any over-the-counter products that are compatible or available for her to use?

JD: There are several great shampoos and conditioners that I recommend to my patients. Many of them are formulated with African-American women in mind, but can work just as well for straight-haired women who have curly perms.

As for conditioners, a woman should look for one that has a high level of protein. (Protein penetrates the hair shaft and gives the hair shine.) Protein conditioners can be used up to four times a month (assuming you're conditioning your hair once a week).

One treatment that I highly recommend to my patients with dry or damaged hair is a reconstructor done once a month. Reconstructors are deep-penetrating protein treatments that are done by professional stylists. (Often the best "treatment" I can offer a particular patient is to refer her to a stylist who is experienced in administering this treatment and recognizes what's best for my patient's type of hair.)

D: What are some myths about hair, ethnic hair in particular?

JD: There are so many! Here are some of my favorites:

i. "Asian women (with their straight hair) can't use products formulated for African-American women (with their curly-kinky hair)." That is so untrue. Any product that does the job is right for any type of hair. Instead of succumbing to niche marketing ploys, ask yourself some basic questions after trying out a product: Does my hair feel stripped? Is it soft? Is it beautiful to look at or to touch? Does my hair appear dull? Let your hair educate you as to what works best.

ii. "Only African-American women perm their hair to 'unkink' it." On the contrary, many ethnic women, for instance, Jewish, Dominican, and Greek, perm their hair, too, for many of the same reasons African-American women do. Some women like the way kinky hair looks when it's been permed.

iii. "All African-American women need to perm their hair, because if they don't they will suffer permanent damage and the hair won't grow." Permed hair is still the preferred style for many African-American women, but it has never been a necessity. The proliferation of Afros and dreadlocks (now called *locks* because of the negative connotations associated with the word *dread*) are proof otherwise.

iv. "African-American women's scalps must be oiled." On the contrary, oiling the scalp with petroleum-based products doesn't do anything beneficial and, in fact, may be counterproductive. It can lead to oil buildup, clogged pores, and hair that gets dirtier faster. I usually recommend that a lightweight oil be applied directly to the hair shaft if the patient has very dry hair.

v. "Castor oil will make your hair grow." Sorry to all of you who've had one spoonful too many growing up! Hair growth is determined by genetics and nutrition. You can drink gallons of castor oil, but if you're not genetically programmed for long hair, it just ain't going to happen because hair length is a function of your *anagen* (growth) cycle. That cycle can vary from six months to ten years. The longer your cycle, the longer your hair *can* become. That's why even twins, if they get their hair cut on the same day, will show different rates of growth (all other things being equal). It's proper diet and care that permit a woman to grow her hair longer. It's genetics that ultimately determines whether that "longer" is to the shoulders or, say, to the waistline.

vi.   "My hair is not growing." Hair is a living thing and is growing all the time. To be more precise about it, the hair on your head is in one of three phases at any given time. There is the *anagen* (growth) phase. Eighty-five percent of the hair on your head is in this phase. There is the *catagen* (resting) phase, which involves about 5 percent of your hair. Finally, there is the *telogen* (shedding) phase, which involves about 10 percent of your hair. As you see, most of the time most of your hair is growing. If it seems as if it isn't, it may be that you are breaking your hair off—because of how you're treating it—just as fast as it is growing. That can happen as a result of vigorous scratching, overperming, dyeing hair too frequently, too much heat application to the hair shaft, and not conditioning hair often enough.

vii.   "Scratching and oiling the scalp are absolutely necessary to get the hair to grow." Nothing could be further from the truth. Scratching the scalp, either with fingers or a comb, contributes to hair breakage. And oiling the scalp, by which most women think of applying petroleum jelly–based products directly on the skin, is also counterproductive. It leads to a buildup of dead skin cells, which clogs the pores.

   If the scalp itches, don't scratch, but do apply a bit of light essential oil to it. Vigorous scratching or combing is usually a self-therapeutic approach to some bothersome conditions such as dandruff, a *fungus,* a burned scalp, etc., which should be medically treated.

D: How does pregnancy affect the hair and scalp?

JD: The hormonal flux that accompanies pregnancy affects women and their hair in a variety of ways. For some women, pregnancy will be a time of great hair growth, where the hair becomes thicker and in general looks better, or a long-standing dandruff problem may be alleviated. For other women, the hormonal flux ushers in a period of increased dandruff, increased hair loss, or the hair becoming more brittle. It just depends. The fact that during pregnancy a woman can experience wholly opposite effects on her hair contradicts the old wives' tale concerning hair loss during pregnancy. Hair loss while pregnant may sometimes have more to do with the general health of the mother-to-be than the pregnancy itself. If your hair is suffering injurious effects during pregnancy, it may be a symptom of an underlying nutritional problem and should be addressed by a health professional.

D: Are there certain treatments that shouldn't be used by pregnant women?

JD: Standard medical logic is that you can dye your hair, assuming you understand the risk, no more than once every three months during pregnancy. Here's how we explain it: That amount of dyeing during pregnancy is equivalent to smoking two cigarettes a year. *I am not stating that it is safe or appropriate to dye your hair during pregnancy. This is a personal decision that each woman must make herself.* Some may choose this risk;

others will decide to defer the risk until after delivery and breast-feeding.

You might also ask, what about chemical straighteners? I would say that the risks are similar to those of dyeing one's hair, simply because we're talking about the use of chemicals on and in the body. However, I'm not aware of any medical literature on the safety of or risks involved with using chemical relaxers during pregnancy. As far as I know there have been no double-blind, controlled studies done as there were with hair dye, smoking, alcohol, and stress. So, while I have addressed this in terms of special concerns for pregnant women, what's most important is that each woman assess her situation and make her own determination. A woman can consider factors—the number of times she would have her hair relaxed during her pregnancy, for instance—and come to her own conclusions. *Even so, I'm not suggesting that chemical relaxers are safe. There is still a risk, however small.*

In general, I'd recommend, at least during the course of your pregnancy, that you refrain from experiments with any new products or nonessential treatments. This is particularly important because of the additives in non-USA made products. (They can contain steroids, mercury, and other potentially harmful chemicals and additives.)

D: Should women with kinky or curly hair care for their hair differently than women with straight or wavy hair?

JD: My rule of thumb for good maintenance of curly or kinky

hair is: more moisture, less heat! Deep conditioning with every shampoo should become part of your standard operating procedure. Be prudent with such techniques as blow-drying, curling the hair with a curling iron, and thermal straightening. Some women press their hair or blow-dry it daily because they want it "just right." It gives them confidence when their hair is looking its best. But, over the long haul, there's a price to be paid. These techniques are all heat-intensive processes that are hard on the hair, and should be used as little as possible.

D: How often should the hair and scalp be cleaned?

JD: Depending on your lifestyle an interval of once every few days to once a week between shampoos is highly recommended. However, if you are a swimmer, or a serious athlete, more frequent shampooing is a necessity. If that's the case, it should always be followed by a deep-conditioning treatment.

D: If a patient of yours wanted to get her hair done by a stylist, what types of salon services should be avoided when treating scalp and hair problems?

JD: Common sense dictates that a woman should avoid any style or treatment that may exacerbate her medical condition. For my psoriasis patients, I counsel them not to begin locking their hair while they're being treated. That's because part of the treatment regimen requires that the scalp be washed at least two times per week, making it impossible to successfully lock hair. In general, when a woman is being treated for any scalp disorders, I ask her not to do anything drastic with her hair. Treatments can run for months, sometimes even a year, and what her hair can take at the beginning of treatment may not be the same at a later point.

To help make a decision about what's possible, I often refer my patients to a stylist/trichologist. I also strongly recommend that a woman get two recommendations from folks with hair similar to her own, in choosing a stylist. That's a good confidence builder in that you know you'll be dealing with someone who understands your needs.

Diseases and Conditions of the Scalp and Hair

D: What diseases and conditions do you encounter in your practice, and what causes them? What treatments are available for your patients? How long does it take to treat various diseases and conditions of the hair and scalp?

JD: As a dermatologist, patients come to me for *alopecia areata,* which are coin-shaped patches of baldness. This condition may occur on the scalp, eyebrows, eyelashes, beard, pubic hair, underarms, and legs. The causes of alopecia areata are stress; or autoimmune problems, e.g., complications of the thyroid; or a family history of diabetes. Whatever the cause, this condition needs to be professionally monitored and treated. When a patient is diagnosed with stress-related alopecia areata, the standard treatment is low-dose injections of steroids once a month for six to twelve months. I warn my patients that the treatment cannot succeed if the source of stress is not addressed. Incorporating exercise into one's life may be as important as steroids to a successful treatment outcome. That's one of the reasons the treatment doesn't go beyond twelve months. If underlying causes are not addressed, no amount of time with a topical or injectable steroid treatment is going to overcome the condition. Untreated or unsuccessfully treated bald patches or "coins" can get larger. The extreme example of this is the condition of *alopecia totalis* or *universalis,* which is the complete absence of body hair. Fortunately, most cases do not become this severe.

Additionally, patients come to me with scalp *fungus.* Many people self-treat the scaly, flaky, sometimes pus-filled patches with dandruff shampoo, thinking it is dandruff. Instead, what they have is a fungus that can be caused by the use of unclean combs and brushes. (However, fungus can have other sources. It can live on inanimate objects such as dirty bed linen and dirty movie theater seats. And our beloved house pets can be fungus carriers, too.) If a microscopic slide review determines fungus, standard treatment is the use of oral antifungal medication, topical creams, and shampoos. Depending on the severity of the case, fungus can usually be eradicated in approximately two to three months. The severe forms of fungus may cause small areas with scarring after everything is healed.

Dandruff, or *seborrheic dermatitis,* is a condition that can affect not only the scalp but also the ears and face. There are many causes of dandruff, including stress, weather changes, and hormonal fluctuations (as in pregnancy). African-Americans have a genetic predisposition to dandruff. Whatever the cause, standard treatment is an over-the-counter topical solution of Nizoral AD 1% (Ketoconazole) and T-Gel (coal tar) or T-Sal (with salicylic acid) shampoos. If Nizoral AD 1% isn't effective, a prescribed 2-percent solution of Nizoral is recommended, or Capex, a steroid-based shampoo. For some cases of dandruff, topical steroid foams such as Luxiq or Olux are used; and there are people who use an overnight application of Derma-smoothe/FS scalp treatment, a peanut-oil and steroid-based medication. Seborrheic dermatitis comes and goes, but it can be controlled. However, it's usually not possible to completely eradicate the condition.

Scalp *psoriasis* appears as thick, silvery plaques. It is a condition determined by family history that plagues 4 percent of Americans. Psoriasis can be treated with the same therapies and medications used for seborrheic dermatitis. For more troublesome cases that don't respond to the above regimen, I may now prescribe Soritane. A person under my care using Soritane must have monthly blood work done. When in treatment, a patient cannot consume any alcohol *at all.* That includes amounts as small as those used in cough medicine.

This medication may not be appropriate for many psoriasis sufferers. For instance, female patients should not be or become pregnant during treatment and *up to 3 years after treatment ends.* Because of the medical and ethical issues involved if a patient gets pregnant, I generally do not prescribe Soritane for my female patients of childbearing age.

Psoriasis is never completely eradicated. It responds variably to topical and oral medications. Treatment is used every time a patient has a flare-up.

D: If you have psoriasis, or seborrheic dermatitis, are you restricted in what you can do with your hair?

JD: Yes, in the sense that these medical conditions need to be treated and monitored before a sensible woman should even think about perming or coloring her hair. Even for someone with a healthy scalp, perming and coloring must be done carefully because it can lead to hair and scalp damage.

D: Do you recommend Rogaine to people with thinning hair? What's the standard treatment for hair loss?

JD: Of course I do, but a person should consult with a dermatologist to detect any underlying medical conditions that may be causing hair loss or thinning. Conditions such as anemia, diabetes, or thyroid problems need to be addressed first before hair transplants or topical replacement therapy are begun. Genetic factors need to be determined or ruled out. Both preexisting medical conditions and genetic factors will have an impact on a person's success (and satisfaction) with the process.

The over-the-counter solutions of Rogaine—2% or 5%—can be used by a woman after checking with her dermatologist. It should be applied twice a day, with a dropper, not a spray, unless you want hair growing out of your forehead or wherever else the spray droplets land. If you are pregnant or nursing, I'd recommend postponing Rogaine until after the baby's born and you've finished nursing. Otherwise, use of Rogaine has minimal side effects—irritation and stinging—which can be addressed if they arise. There is absolutely no need to buy the accompanying shampoo or conditioner. Purchase products that are gentle (after all, you're growing fragile new hair) and you should do just fine.

When my patients ask me how long it will take, in other words, how long they must be on a Rogaine regimen, my considered reply is "as long as it's important to you." At the very least, 50 percent of Rogaine users will decrease the amount of hair being shed, and 50 percent of users will both decrease shedding and be able to regrow *some* lost hair.

Propecia is an excellent oral medication for male-pattern baldness in men, and is used in conjunction with Rogaine. Even though male-pattern baldness is found in women these days, I don't recommend Propecia for my women patients. It hasn't been shown to be particularly successful, and studies have shown that it can harm fetuses.

D: Are transplants and other hair replacement therapies a viable option for everyone?

JD: Hair transplants are effective, but they are both expensive and complicated. It is best to get references before choosing a dermatologist or a plastic surgeon to perform the procedure. To ensure the best results, a person should adhere religiously to her postop instructions and, as in using Rogaine, should practice gentle hair care. I do caution against getting hair transplants if you are a keloid-prone person. (Keloids are raised, thickened, flesh-colored scars.)

D: What exactly does a transplant involve?

JD: In terms of hair transplants, what a dermatologist does is take a patch of hair from the back of the patient's scalp, which, even for male patients with significant U-shaped baldness, is still the thickest part of one's hair. We call this section the "harvest area." That patch is cut into tiny pieces containing one to two hair follicles, and stored in a petri dish of saline solution. The next step in the procedure is the *microscopic hair transplantation* itself. The dermatologist inserts the follicle pieces (you may have heard them referred to as "plugs," a term I don't care for) into slits cut into the front (anterior) of the patient's scalp, or wherever the patient wants her or his hair to be restored. (The necessity of making incisions is why hair transplants aren't a viable option for keloid-prone folks. The kind of scarring produced wouldn't allow the follicle pieces to "take" to the scalp.) All of this, which can take up to five or six hours and involves an average of five hundred separate transplantations, is serious business. It's a bloody process, and when the dermatologist is done the scalp is bandaged (although there are no stitches involved).

Remember I mentioned the importance of following postoperative instructions? Here's what a patient will have to do: start on a regimen of prednisone (an anti-inflammatory drug) and an antibiotic, such as Keflex or Omnicef. In addition to the medications, a person will need to sleep virtually upright for the first two nights after the procedure, and refrain from washing her or his scalp for seven to ten days.

I might add that sometimes a single hair transplant isn't sufficient, and that a person will have to have an additional three to four sessions spaced out over two-month intervals.

Finally, and this is another reason I don't consider hair transplants a magic solution, each session can cost a person upward of $10,000. You can do the math.

The long and the short of it is that hair transplants are not for the squeamish, the keloid prone, or the poor!

D: Does a woman's hair always have to fall out if she is on chemotherapy? How do you treat women who are undergoing chemotherapy?

JD: Most people receiving chemotherapy lose their hair, but not all people receiving chemotherapy do. Truth be told, the latter is a small group (approximately 20 percent of all patients).

Chemotherapy works by killing rapidly dividing cells—and while its target is cancer cells, it kills any other rapidly dividing cells such as, you guessed it, hair cells. Therefore, the resting and shedding phases described before in the normal cycle of hair growth are accelerated and more pronounced. Hence the hair loss. I reassure my patients that their hair can and will grow back. If I can help them see that an acute but temporary hair loss is a small price to pay for a prolonged life, it helps put things in perspective. Patience and a great wig are the best medicine in this case.

D: What is the leading cause of hair loss among women? Among women of color?

JD: I would say that two of the leading causes of hair loss among women are perming and coloring the hair, particularly if they're not done by a competent beautician or stylist. Overdoing those styling treatments, and glue residue from extensions and weaves, can lead to *follicular degeneration syndrome*. The syndrome can be diagnosed in an office visit, in which we conduct a hair pull test, examine hair microscopically, and perform a scalp biopsy.

   Traction alopecia is caused by hair that is pulled very tightly. Many a woman grew up with elaborately braided or twisted hair held in place by barrettes or elastic bands. Years later, her childhood hairdo can be deduced because of her sparse hairline. The same holds true of women who constantly wear their hair tightly braided or twisted. Sooner or later you will lose hair. Once traction alopecia has occurred, the virgin hairline can never be restored.

Unfortunately, one of the easiest conditions for me to diagnose is *trichotillomania*. Every time a woman comes into my office looking like she cuts her own hair with hedge clippers, I think to myself, "Uh-oh, trichotillomania." This stress-induced condition is caused by a person actually pulling out patches of her own hair. Trichotillomania occurs in people of all ages. Sadly, it is much more common these days, a by-product of our fast-paced, overbooked lives.

Once the condition is confirmed, I recommend an expert stylist to my patients, but I also advise that they incorporate stress-relieving activities—exercise, hobbies, etc.—into their lives, and, not infrequently, refer them to a mental health professional.

Trichotillomania takes a multifaceted approach to overcome: While I, or another understanding dermatologist, do what I can to treat the hair loss, a stylist does what she or he can to help restore a patient's hair to health. Often we counsel the patient about hair-care techniques in order to prevent further damage. (Many times patients, in desperation, resort to masking hairdos such as wigs, weaves, or extensions. These, when not used properly, can cause even more damage to the hair and scalp.) However, our best efforts won't be sufficient if the patient doesn't get some therapeutic counsel for whatever it is that is causing her so much stress that she is literally tearing her hair out.

Hair loss is sometimes a symptom of diseases like *lupus,*

which is why I encourage women who are experiencing hair loss to get a medical consultation, in addition to any discussions with their stylist. A brilliant new hairdo to mask hair loss or thinning is no cure for a serious, undiagnosed disease.

D: What role, if any, does hair dyeing play in hair loss?

JD: If I could convince my patients not to use home coloring kits at all, I'd be a happier dermatologist. But being a pragmatic dermatologist, I counsel them not to color the hair more than once every three months. And, I encourage them to see a professional colorist a minimum of once a year.

D: What role, if any, does hair straightening or perming play in hair loss?

JD: It is no secret that heat and chemicals are hard on both the hair and the scalp. Perms and thermal straightening should be done in moderation and in intervals of six to eight weeks and one to two weeks, respectively. I strongly urge women to have these treatments done by competent professionals. There is nothing inherently wrong with having hair permed or straightened. Under a beautician's care there doesn't have to be any hair loss.

D: What role, if any, do wigs play in hair loss?

JD: Wigs can become a crutch and unfortunately cause a woman to neglect whatever hair she does have on her head. Just because one's own hair and scalp aren't seen in public doesn't mean that they should go for long periods without cleaning and conditioning.

D: Are diseases and subsequent treatment for men and women identical?

JD: In general, yes. However, in the case of male-pattern baldness the choice of pharmaceutical options is more limited for women than it is for men.

D: Do you recommend wigs or extensions to your patients when they are being treated for extreme hair loss or scalp conditions?

JD: With extreme hair loss a wig or extensions are sensible solutions. However, whatever style is adopted, the dermatologist must be able to treat the ongoing medical condition. It's common sense: When your hair and scalp are endangered, that is not the time to apply perms or color, or to adopt high-maintenance hairstyles that can actually interfere with a treatment regimen. After all, these very practices may have contributed to the hair loss in the first place. If a patient wants extensions, I recommend that they be sewn in, not glued. Glue can cause chemical burns and fungal problems on the scalp.

D: Does diet play a role in hair and scalp conditions?

JD: If a woman is on a severe, i.e., a nutritionally dubious diet, that can affect her hair. So, while there are no special diets that will guarantee a woman a beautiful, healthy head of hair, there are some commonsensical things you can do that promote overall good health. I've said it before and I'll say it again: Eating a well-balanced diet, taking a daily multivitamin, and getting exercise to help reduce the effects of stress are your first and best defenses. After all, you are what you eat, and your hair reflects that.

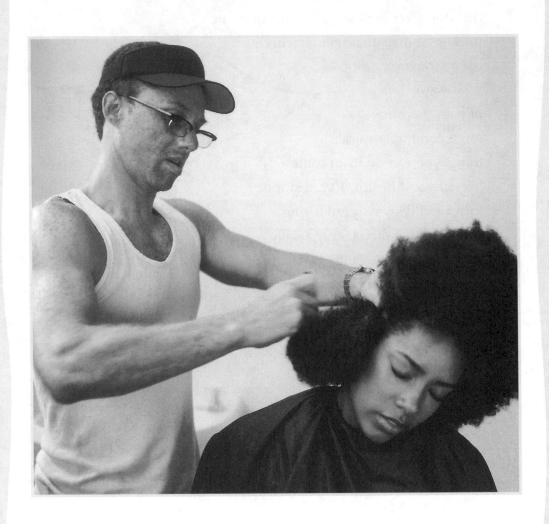

The Sweet "Hairafter"
(an Afterthought)

Hair Rules! came to me as an astounding revelation when I found myself simultaneously immersed in two worlds. One world, that of the constantly changing, competitive fashion industry, which has dictated the trends in both music and film in the last ten years, and the second, a salon world where clients range from 9-to-9 Wall Street executives to celebrities to stay-at-home moms. Somehow I've managed to balance my salon obligations with a sometimes hectic freelance schedule. I'm often called at the eleventh hour to revamp and restore the hair of people who simply cannot afford to have a bad hair day.

In my work I started to see a parallel between the needs of my high-profile clients, with their access to the very best, and the needs of the working girl. Across the board there is now a large demand for information on how to care for hair other than straight hair. Nonstraight hair, ranging from kinky to wavy, has only recently become "respectable" rather than assigned to be covered up and disguised. Whether kinky, curly, or wavy, the assault on nonstraight hair's various textures, whether from ignorance or lack of positive imagery, has subsided. Now more than ever, women want to know how to care for and style it properly.

From the very beginning, I didn't want *Hair Rules!* simply to be a book with some glamorous photos and unrealistic images of hair on models that would intimidate my reader. Why would I want to falsely depict hairstyles that only a pro could pull off? None of the natural textures featured in this book were overstyled with heat or any other tool or process that might mislead a reader into believing she could achieve the same effect with her own hair. My models were carefully selected based on their hair type, so that the reader's own hair type would be recognized (and represented) on an honest, positive tip.

Really, writing this book has been my attempt to say that nonstraight hair is beautiful and unique. Yes, it presents its care challenges, but they can be met. My philosophy was and always has been to respect women's hair, and glorify it by working with it, not against it. Lately, I've seen a lot of beautiful heads of kinky, curly, and extremely wavy hair strutting around these streets. If the advice and information in *Hair Rules!* can help add one more beautiful head of hair to the parade, I'll feel that I accomplished what I set out to do.

Acknowledgments

I've been on a mission. The result has been this book. Nothing as complex as this happens, however, without the support and generosity of family, friends, and colleagues. I'd like to thank all the many folks who helped me have my say:

Thank you Jesus, my family (who were right there when I needed them), Ann T. Greene, Gregg Hubbard, Jeanine B. Downie, MD, Louis Licari, Tomiko Fraser, Marc and Jenny Baptiste, Jeffrey Fulvimar, Crawford Morgan, Pauline St. Denis, Mezz Assef and Sun West Studios, Kara Young, Susan Carmen, Tracy Murphy, Robin Page, Candice Dhakhwa, Wendy Graham, Annette Rosario, Elisabet Davidsdottir, Minnie Driver, Sarah Jessica Parker, Amoy, Kiara, Carlos Taylor, Carla Gentry, Reny Monk, Gioietta Vitale, Carlotta Jacobson, Santa Polanco and Erica Szabo of Louis Licari Salon, Neal Hamil and Charlotte Wagster of the Ford Model Agency, Tahlani Knights and Ashton Hundley of Qmodels, Anna Shinderovsky and Joyce Mills of CMI, Enid Shore, Kim Brown, Stephanie Latham, Carla Nugent, Tasha Turner of *VIBE* magazine, Leigh Rossini, and the staff of Louis Licari Salon.

Also a special thank-you to all the photographers whose work I've had the pleasure of contributing to over the years:

Ellen von Un Werth, Marc Baptiste, Sante D'Orazio, Walter Chin, Ricardo Tinneli, Pauline St. Denis, Christian Witkin, Arnaldo Anaya-Lucca, Arthur Elgort, and Dah Len.

A special thank-you to Ricky's Cosmetics of New York City.

And for helping me get my word out to the world, thank you to Tracey Gardner and Michael Bourret at Jane Dystel Literary Management, and Melody Guy at Villard, Random House.

Creative direction for *Hair Rules!* is by Marc Baptiste.
Illustrations by Jeffrey Fulvimar.
Photo (Chapter 4) is by Ellen von Un Werth.
Still life by Pauline St. Denis.
Weaves by Carla Gentry.
Color by Louis Licari.

Check out the website for more information: www.HairRules.com.